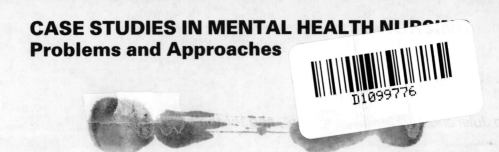

CASE STUDIES IN MENTAL HEALTH NURSING
Problems and Approaches

CASE STUDIES IN MENTAL HEALTH NURSING
Problems and Approaches

To Julia and Lynne for being here, and for their understanding.

CASE STUDIES IN MENTAL HEALTH NURSING
Problems and Approaches

Keith Briggs

RMN DN(Lond) Cert Ed RNT
Nurse Tutor at High Royds Hospital, Menston, West Yorkshire;
Chairman of the Board of Examiners for Mental Nursing

Andrew Stewart

RMN RGN DN(Lond) Cert Ed RNT
Senior Tutor at Scalebor Park Hospital, Burley-in-Wharfedale,
West Yorkshire; Member of the Panel of Examiners for Mental
Nursing

Churchill Livingstone ▦

EDINBURGH LONDON MELBOURNE AND NEW YORK 1987

CHURCHILL LIVINGSTONE
Medical Division of Longman Group UK Limited

Distributed in the United States of America by Churchill
Livingstone Inc., 1560 Broadway, New York, N.Y. 10036,
and by associated companies, branches and
representatives throughout the world.

First published 1987
  Reprinted 1988
  Reprinted 1989

ISBN   0-443-03570-9

British Library Cataloguing in Publication Data
Briggs, Keith
  Case studies in mental health nursing:
  problems and approaches.
  1. Psychiatric nursing — Problems,
  exercises, etc.
  I. Title   II. Stewart, Andrew
  610.73'68'076   RC440

Library of Congress Cataloging in Publication Data
Briggs, Keith.
  Case studies in mental health nursing.
  1. Psychiatric nursing — Case studies.
2. Psychiatric nursing — Examinations, questions, etc.
I. Stewart, Andrew (K. Andrew)   II. Title.
[DNLM: 1. Psychiatric Nursing. WY 160 B854c]
RC440.B67   1987   610.73'68   86-26906

Produced by Longman Singapore Publishers (Pte) Ltd.
Printed in Singapore

Introduction

Acknowledgeme

This book is written mainly for students studying for part III of the Register (Registered Mental Nurse) but will also prove useful for those undertaking Enrolled Nurse (Mental) training. It should also prove to be of value to tutors as a teaching aid for both individual and group sessions.

In content the book covers a wide range of psychiatric problems from a nursing perspective, using fictitious case studies. The cases describe clients who exhibit difficulties which are familiar to nursing staff and require nursing interventions which are based on sound principles. The nurse is considered to have a therapeutic function in his or her own right, acting as a facilitator of change. The relationship between nurse and client is seen as dynamic and interactive.

How to use this book

There are 13 sections to the book. Each starts with a case study around which a number of questions are posed. Nine multiple choice questions follow the case study and are directly linked to it. A full analysis of each question is undertaken and individual items are discussed with a rationale for the final choice. Three structured essay questions follow which are constructed around the same case. A specimen answer is given for the first of these questions and answer guides given for the other two.

We see the book as a text which enables the student to become actively involved in the learning process. In answering the multiple choice questions, problems have to be solved and decisions made by comparing the information given in each item and making choices based on that evaluation. The majority of questions are concerned with the application of knowledge rather than the recall of facts. Immediate feedback can be obtained by comparing the choice made with the rationale given. The discussion of each answer can help students to develop their understanding of the problem. Students are further invited to construct written answers to the structured questions and to compare the outcomes with the specimen answer and answer guides.

Marking of the multiple choice questions is easy as we believe there is only one correct answer. The value of the book, however, does not simply lie in making correct choices but more in the discussions around the questions. The specimen answer and answer guides are intended to give the student some indication of expected content in the written areas.

Although the book can be read, cover to cover, and contains a lot of psychiatric nursing knowledge, we advise a more participative approach in which the student makes attempts at all of the questions. In this way the text can be used to review or increase knowledge on a step by step basis as the student comes into contact with particular types of client.

K. B.
A. S.

Acknowledgements

We would like to express our sincere thanks to all of the students who offered many useful comments regarding the composition of this book, and to Michelle Collins for giving up her time in helping to type the script.

Contents

Contents

1. The experience of admission and its effects

Adrian Mullet is 42 years old. He has been married to Shirley for 19 years and they have two children, Mark aged 14, and Nicola aged 11.

On leaving school Adrian started work in a large department store. Since that time he has progressed through the management structure of the company and is now head of the buying section.

Adrian has never experienced difficulties in forming relationships. He and his wife have a varied and active social life both independently and jointly.

Since gaining promotion 1 year ago he has gradually developed feelings of inadequacy, doubting his abilities and finding difficulty in making decisions. His immediate manager has assured him that there is nothing wrong with his work. Despite these assurances he finds himself unable to stop worrying.

Adrian was treated by his general practitioner for 3 months before being referred to a consultant psychiatrist. Following the consultation he agreed to admission for assessment and is at present resident on an integrated acute ward within a large psychiatric hospital.

Multiple choice questions

1. Which one of the following groups contains a sequence of actions which would be effective in responding to Adrian's anxiety about admission?
   A Assess the cause, orientate to the area and offer explanations.
   B Orientate to the area, offer explanations and ensure physical contact.
   C Offer explanations, ensure physical contact and assess the cause.
   D Ensure physical contact, assess the cause and orientate to the area.

2. Which one of the following groups contains strategies which would all form part of a nursing assessment?
   A Collection of data, recording of observations and identification of goals.
   B Recording of observations, identification of goals and interviewing of client.
   C Identification of goals, interviewing of client and collection of data.
   D Interviewing of client, collection of data and recording of observations.

3. Which one of the following would be the most appropriate response for the nurse to make if Adrian states, 'I don't know how my family will manage, I have always taken care of things at home?'
   A Acknowledge the concerns and feelings he is expressing and suggest discussing available options.
   B Explain to him that he will not be in hospital long and that he is not going to help his family by worrying.
   C Reassure him that his family will manage because people are always more capable than they are given credit for.
   D Suggest that he concentrates on getting better and let other people worry about helping his family.

4. Which one of the following groups contains factors which would all lead to adoption of the sick role?
   A Reduce involvement in the decision-making process, ensure that Adrian is orientated to the ward environment and limit the information given to that which is necessary.
   B Ensure that Adrian is orientated to the ward environment, limit the information given to that which is necessary and ensure that rules and policies are adhered to.
   C Limit the information given to that which is necessary, ensure that rules and policies are adhered to and reduce involvement in the decision-making process.
   D Ensure that rules and policies are adhered to, reduce involvement in the decision-making process and ensure that Adrian is orientated to the ward environment.

5. Which one of the following offers the best explanation for Adrian reacting in a frightened, defensive manner during the process of admission? Because he:
   A feels that too many questions of a personal nature are being asked.
   B misinterprets stimuli due to his state of heightened arousal.
   C feels that he does not really need to be in hospital.
   D believes that he should be seen by a doctor not a nurse.

6. Which one of the following groups contains tasks which are all the responsibility of the nurse whilst admitting Adrian to the ward?
   A Accurate documentation, ensuring access to a doctor and maintaining safety of personal property.
   B Ensuring access to a doctor, maintaining safety of personal property and explanation of personal rights.
   C Maintaining safety of personal property, explanation of personal rights and accurate documentation.
   D Explanation of personal rights, accurate documentation and ensuring access to a doctor.

7. Which one of the following groups contains skills which would all be appropriate for the nurse to use when interviewing Adrian at the time of admission?
   A Organising the setting, listening and attending, and judging the duration of the interview.
   B Listening and attending, judging the duration of the interview and analysing the data.
   C Judging the duration of the interview, analysing the data and organising the setting.
   D Analysing the data, organising the setting, and listening and attending.

8. Which one of the following groups contains emotions which may all be experienced by Adrian's wife upon his admission?
   A Anger, emotional bonding and rejection.
   B Emotional bonding, rejection and guilt.
   C Rejection, guilt and anger.
   D Guilt, anger and emotional bonding.

9. Which one of the following is the most appropriate verbal response for the nurse to make when, during the admission interviews, Adrian's wife asks, 'How long do you think Adrian will have to stay in hospital?'
   A 'This is difficult to say at the moment, perhaps we could discuss it again after we have had a chance to work with Adrian for a while.'
   B 'I can see that you are worried and I understand that. However this is the sort of issue you should take up with the doctor.'
   C 'Perhaps we can discuss this later, I would like to finish this initial interview and I am sure Adrian has enough to think about at the moment.'
   D 'For us to be able to help Adrian come to terms with his problems effectively I would say he needs to be here for a period of 4 to 6 weeks.'

Answer keys to MCQs

1. The process of admission to hospital is one which creates a great deal of anxiety for most individuals. The reasons are numerous, but it is the responsibility of the nurse to allay anxiety as effectively as possible.

    Option A is the correct response. The initial action would be an attempt by the nurse to ascertain the cause of a person's anxiety. When this has been achieved, appropriate interventions could be employed. Such measures could include familiarising the individual with the environment and attempting to reduce uncertainty by answering as many questions as possible.

    Options B, C, and D: All include making physical contact with the individual. This may be an acceptable strategy but it must be remembered that the person is anxious and is likely to be in an aroused state. Under circumstances such as this, physical contact can be misinterpreted, and if it is not carried out with sensitivity and skill, can increase rather than decrease anxiety.

2. Assessment of a person's needs or problems is a complex and multifactorial aspect of nursing. The purpose of such an assessment is to gain a picture of the person which is as complete as possible.

    Option D is the correct response: interviewing the client and significant people in his life to clarify their perceptions, expectations and personal details; observing actions, interactions and life abilities; collecting relevant data such as reports compiled by other health workers. All of these processes form part of a nursing assessment.

    Options A, B and C: All contain the proposal that identifying goals is a part of nursing assessment. It is an essential part of the care process but is more associated with the planning of care, which would follow a careful and comprehensive assessment.

3. Many people who are experiencing the necessity of admission are plagued with concerns, not only about themselves but also the situation in which they feel they have left their families. The skilled nurse should recognise that such feelings may be borne out of a person's desire to be missed or wanted by his family, but are nevertheless real.

    Option A is the correct response in that the feelings which Adrian is expressing are accepted by the nurse. It is important, however, that the nurse does not foster the development of dependency in Adrian. This can be avoided by acknowledging the reality of his concerns and offering to help him examine the available options.

Options B, C and D: are all pacifying statements which do nothing to help Adrian with his real concerns. In addition, such responses are likely to interfere with the formation of effective relationships by suggesting to Adrian that the nurse is not really concerned with helping, but more in deflecting a difficult statement.

4. The experience of admission can be depersonalising to a client. Nursing staff and the hospital itself play their part in this process by attitudes, actions, approaches and organisational policies. Such an experience may result in a person developing an outlook which is referred to as the 'sick role'.

    With a perception such as this Adrian would believe, 'I am sick, you are the helpers'. Nursing care would be more concerned with doing to, rather than doing with; and the whole atmosphere would foster dependence rather than independence.

    Option C is the correct response. Each of these actions would reduce Adrian's involvement in his care and thereby decrease his independence.

    Options A, B and D: All include orientation to the ward environment. In itself this would not foster the development of the sick role.

5. At this time Adrian will be experiencing a mixture of emotions. The most common reactions are likely to be those of anxiety and concern. When such feelings occur the body is automatically placed in a state of readiness: the fight or flight response. Due to the release of the hormone adrenalin, specific physiological changes occur. There is also a change in the individual's level of arousal and this increases the chances of stimuli being misinterpreted.

    Option B is therefore the correct response.

    Option A   Questions of a personal nature may result in Adrian becoming irritated and to some extent defensive; however they are unlikely to provoke a reaction of fear.

    Options C and D: The feelings and reactions associated with such beliefs are more likely to be those of resentment and resignation, rather than fear and defensiveness.

6. During the process of admission the nurse has specific responsibilities. The process of nursing assessment will be commenced. The requirement for maintaining the dignity and as far as possible the independence of the individual is of the utmost importance. Additionally, the person who is being admitted will expect that any property which he has placed into the hands of the nurse will be kept in safety.

    Option C is the correct response. All of the factors concerned are the responsibility of the nurse.

Options A, B and D: All suggest that the nurse should ensure access to a medical officer, which is one of the rights of the patient. The nurse should contact the doctor as soon as possible after admission. Unlike the other responsibilities, however, it is not something which the nurse can either directly control or ensure.

7. One aspect of a nursing assessment is the conduction of interviews with Adrian, and also with those who are significant in his life. During the interviews a great deal of information can be obtained. This would include the individual's perception of the problem, and the expectations of both Adrian and his family. In order to maximise the benefit of the interviews they should be conducted in a manner which is both sensitive and skilful.

Option A is the correct response. The nurse must have due regard for the setting of the interview and try to create an atmosphere of relaxation and security. During the actual interview she should demonstrate her concern, interest and involvement. Such an interview may release a variety of emotions in Adrian: the nurse should therefore be able to assess the optimum duration of the interview and skilfully conclude the session when appropriate.

Options B, C and D: All include the analysis of data. This is an essential part of the process of care planning, but would not form part of the skill repertoire of the nurse during interview sessions.

8. When one member of a family is admitted to hospital it has a profound effect on the dynamics of the family unit and also on the emotions of individual members.
    Adrian has managed many of the financial and maintenance functions of the household. His wife may now feel abandoned and uncertain of the effects of Adrian's hospitalisation on the rest of the family. Remorse, guilt and a degree of hostility may be experienced by Mrs Mullet. These feelings may be displaced onto Adrian, the children, or the hospital and its staff.

Option C is the correct response.

Options A, B and D: All contain the process of emotional bonding. This is unlikely to occur in relation to his need for admission. If it does occur it is likely to be at a later stage when the family experience a feeling of being closer to each other than before, because of their experiences.

9. Such questions, posed to nursing staff, are both common and valid. The nurse must not respond with platitudes, or lie, or give false hope. These are all responses which emanate from the nurse's lack of interest in the individual, or are attempts to resolve her own anxiety in the situation. Her approach should be one which deals with the question in an honest and mature manner.

Option A is the correct response. The nurse is being honest in that it is impossible to say how long Adrian will be in hospital. It is possible, based on experience, to estimate an average length of stay but a more appropriate response would be to discuss the matter again following a comprehensive assessment of Adrian's needs.

Option B recognises the concerns which Adrian's wife feels but then 'passes the buck' to someone else. Her concerns are real and immediate which is why she has asked the question. It may be appropriate at a later stage to call in a member of the medical staff but only if Adrians' wife is not satisfied with the response of the nurse.

Option C will not help Adrian or his wife. Such a response may irritate Adrian or make him feel guilty. At the same time it is effectively saying to Adrian's wife; 'Your concerns are of little consequence'.

Option D: As indicated in the answer to option A, an estimate such as this may be made, based on experience. It is not, however, the most appropriate response.

Essay questions

1. Adrian Mullet is head of the buying department in a large store. For the past 12 months he has been experiencing feelings of self-doubt and inadequacy. He has recently agreed to in-patient care for a period of assessment. He has been admitted to an integrated acute unit in a large local psychiatric hospital.

   A Describe the feelings which Adrian may experience as a result of this admission.   25%

   B Indicate some common behaviours which are associated with these feelings.   25%

   C Describe nursing interventions which may help to prevent or resolve these feelings related to admission.   50%

2. Adrian Mullet is married with two children. He holds a responsible position as head of a department in a large local store.

   He has recently been admitted to a mixed-sex acute unit for a period of assessment because of long-standing feelings of inadequacy and doubts about his abilities.

   A Outline those factors which contribute to the development of the sick role.   25%

   B Describe the behaviours which may result when an individual moves into the sick role.   25%

   C Describe nursing interventions and approaches which would reduce the risk of an individual adopting the sick role.   50%

3. Adrian Mullet is 42 years old, married and has two children aged 14 and 11 years.

   Following 12 months of increasing self-doubt and feelings of inadequacy he has been admitted to an integrated acute unit for a period of assessment.

   This is Adrian's first experience of a psychiatric hospital.

   A Discuss the feelings and difficulties which Adrian's wife and children may experience.   40%

   B Describe ways in which the nursing staff can help this family.   60%

[Handwritten margin notes:]

more habits
brashness
withdrawn tearful
restlessness insomnia
anorexia
gastro-intestinal discomfort

Behaviour

interventions — empathise with his feelings
Approach from nurse — calm, quiet, unhurried, friendly.
Explain nurses role

associated with

feelings:
anxiety
insecurity
family worries
guilt
rejection
relief
embarrassment

Specimen answer

1. A The feelings which are experienced will be <u>unique</u> to Adrian. There are, however, certain reactions which are likely to occur in anyone who is in a strange environment, for reasons they cannot fully comprehend.

   Feelings of anxiety will probably be the most common experience. Such anxiety may emanate from a sense of insecurity at being in a new environment, with strange faces and rules. Adrian will be uncertain of what is expected of him; he will have perceptions related to what is happening to him and be concerned about whether he is in any danger. He may also worry about what is happening to his wife and children: How are people treating them? How are they managing?

   It is to be expected that at some time he will feel guilty about leaving his wife and children and wonder whether he could or should have done things differently.

   Ideas of rejection may also occur to him. He may fear that the family will feel better off without him, and perhaps that in a sense they wanted him to be admitted to make things easier for themselves.

   A feeling of relief might be experienced that at last something is being done to help him, and that his problems have been legitimised by being defined as an 'illness'.

   Because he has been admitted to a mixed unit he may experience embarrassment. This ward-based embarrassment may be compounded by the necessity of sleeping in the same room as others. The feeling may also relate to the stigma associated with mental illness and what his friends and neighbours might think and say.

   B The behaviours which may be evident are an increase in habits or mannerisms as a result of feelings of anxiety and insecurity. A brashness or over-compensation may also indicate anxiety or possible embarrassment. Occasionally, Adrian may laugh in a way which appears false and perhaps forced. Alternatively, in response to anxiety he may become quiet and withdrawn.

   Restlessness, a desire to to leave the hospital environment and signs of dependence upon the staff or the system are also indicators that Adrian may be experiencing anxiety.

   Feelings of rejection could present as tearfulness, a desire to leave the hospital and return home, or possibly as expressions of anger and confrontation through the process of displacement. Additionally, a variety of physical disturbances might present as a consequence of anxiety, such as insomnia, anorexia and gastro-intestinal discomfort.

   C On meeting Adrian the nurse must try to empathise with the feelings that he will be experiencing. She should approach him in a calm, quiet, unhurried, friendly yet professional manner. After greeting him by name, she should introduce herself and explain her role in the admission and assessment procedure. Any questions which Adrian asks should be answered as far as

non-judgemental

intervention – *Demonstrate reliability,*
consistency, warmth, honesty.
counselling — *Listen, attending, responding.*
skills

possible and, where relevant, referred to personnel who can supply a more accurate response.

In attempting to develop a trusting relationship, the nurse must demonstrate her reliability, consistency, warmth and honesty. The routines and policies of the unit should be explained and any misconceptions related to expectations, discussed and clarified.

Throughout the process of admission Adrian must be encouraged to be involved in his own care—questions should be answered clearly, concisely and honestly.

The ward environment may be a source of some concern to Adrian. The nurse must try to allay this anxiety by showing him the geography of the unit, with particular reference to sleeping areas and the segregation of male and female toilets and sanitary annexes. In this way he may be helped to feel less threatened by the thoughts of a mixed unit.

The nurse must use counselling skills such as listening, attending, organising and responding in order to encourage Adrian to ventilate his feelings. Ample opportunity has to be given for exploration of these feelings. Some emotional release may be experienced by Adrian whilst he is discussing his anxieties and emotions. This process can be helped by the nurse concerned demonstrating an air of non-judgemental acceptance throughout.

In order to reduce his feelings of rejection the nurse must involve Adrian's family as much as possible in his care. By making herself available to the family, acting as a link person, and asking for their perceptions of the problems, she demonstrates that these are difficulties which the family can work out together.

The nurse should take every opportunity to encourage Adrian to discuss his feelings regarding his home circumstances, utilising things his wife and children may have said as prompts. She should encourage Adrian to keep with him, on his person, or by his bed, small mementoes which act as a link with his family. From an early stage in his care he must be encouraged to discuss his 'life after discharge'; this will help Adrian to maintain clear perceptions of his care plan and intended goals. Through these discussions, areas such as public stigma and the reactions of friends and workmates might be examined.

All of these aspects are important in preventing or resolving the feelings which Adrian may experience. The nurse should remember that the most important part of this process is her use of skills to allow him to identify and ventilate what he is feeling, in order that the most appropriate action might be taken.

Answer guides

2. A Perceptions of client:
       — influenced by culture, class and the media
       — 'I am ill: treat me'
       — status of medical profession
       — power of medical profession
       — need for problems to be legitimised
       — 'I cannot handle responsibility'.
       Perceptions of carers:
       — 'you are ill: I will solve your problems'
       — own status
       — uniforms
       — actions
       — implicit attitudes.
       Role stripping process:
       — removal of day clothes and transfer into night clothes
       — minimisation of possessions
       — reduction of privacy; sharing rooms
       — neglecting family unit and concentrating on the individual.
       Organisational factors:
       — routine
       — policies
       — access to family governed by others
       — need to request permission for many things
       — medical examination
       — issue of sick certificate
       — sickness payments.
    B Abdication of responsibilities:
       — reduced concern for outside events and family circumstances
       — reluctance to become involved in family responsibilities.
       Reduction of personal responsibility:
       — neglect of self
       — subservience to those seen as being in 'authority'.
       Hesitation in decision-making:
       — uncertainty, restlessness
       — increased need for support when making decisions.
       Dependency:
       — reluctance to leave security of hospital environment.
       Conformity:
       — acceptance of what others decide.
    C Education of general public, medical and nursing staff by providing
       information regarding rights, responsibilities and roles.
           Philosophy of carers should be based on a shared responsibility, working

'with' the client rather than on him, incorporating a belief in the uniqueness of the individual.

Encouraging personal identity by the use of clothing, personal possessions and correct forms of address.

Maintain personal dignity by ensuring privacy in all situations.

Encourage client involvement and involvement of family, where possible, in all stages of the care programme.

Promote personal responsibility by asking opinions of, and encouraging decisions by, the client regarding his own care. Plan for discharge and after care at the earliest opportunity—this may be shortly after the initial assessment, during the assessment itself or at the time of admission.

Explanation should be given by the carers regarding their actions or anything which the client wishes to know. This relatively simple strategy encourages, in the individual concerned, the belief that he has a right to know what is happening.

Reduction of routine as much as possible: adopt a more individualised approach to organisational restrictions. Examination of policies which affect the client such as visiting, staff uniforms and client clothing.

3. A The feelings of the family may include:
   — anxiety
   — guilt
   — loneliness
   — rejection
   — relief
   — embarrassment
   — bewilderment
   — anger
   — sadness.
   The difficulties experienced may include:
   Wife:
   — changes in role, the assumption of paternal as well as maternal responsibilities
   — financial: possible loss of, or reduced income combined with increased expenditure on such items as visiting
   — increased workload to maintain the home, and responsibilities to Adrian
   — administrative aspects such as completion of statements, circulars and payment of accounts
   — questions from children which she finds difficult if not impossible to answer
   — loss of company from her husband, loss of physical contact, sexual and psychological needs unfulfilled
   — isolation due to neglect or embarrassment of friends.
   Children:
   — temporary loss of attention due to additional responsibilities of mother

— expectations of others regarding sharing responsibility with mother
— confusion and uncertainty due to change of parental roles
— isolation due to neglect and embarrassment of friends
— ridicule from other children.

B Nursing staff to make themselves available:
  — ensure time for discussion is adequate and appropriate
  — present an approachable personality
  — initiate as well as respond to conversation.

Assist Adrian's wife to ventilate and acknowledge her feelings by:
— organising a conducive setting
— adopting a non-judgemental and encouraging approach
— using open-ended questioning techniques
— using responding skills
— demonstrating acceptance, understanding and a willingness to discuss her feelings and concerns.

Offer support:
— verbally: the use of words or phrases which are encouraging or demonstrate understanding
— non-verbally: a touch, arm around the shoulder, facial expression.

Give explanations as far as possible about what is happening with Adrian, answering any questions or concerns regarding policies or care.

Encourage involvement of the family in Adrian's care programme: such aspects as initial problems, goals and ongoing problems can all be discussed.

Provide help and support for Mrs Mullet related to the ongoing needs of her children. Their need for support, security, attention and information should all be assessed and wherever necessary strategies examined.

Arrange contact with social work agencies, and provide an explanation of their roles and ways in which assistance may be available to help the family, e.g., home helps, financial assistance.

Assist in the maintenance of family contacts; assess visiting and leave opportunities; reduce organisational difficulties as much as possible.

2. The anxiety response as a disturbed coping pattern

Gwen Seymour is a 35-year-old married woman with two children, a daughter aged 13 and a son of 11.

At school she was described as 'highly strung' and whilst quite bright academically she always doubted her own abilities. When she was around 12 years of age, there was a period of time when she refused to go to school. This was associated with a change of area. She married, at the age of 20, and left work shortly afterwards to start a family.

Over the last few years she has experienced increasing anxiety about leaving the home. At present she is virtually housebound and experiences attacks of severe panic if the need to go outside the house arises.

Her husband, John, is finding it difficult to conduct all of the household business as well as remain in employment. She has been referred to the community psychiatric nursing services.

Multiple choice questions

1. Which one of the following gives rise to the physical symptoms of anxiety?
   Overactivity of the:
   A Sympathetic nervous system.
   B Pyramidal nervous system.
   C Parasympathetic nervous system.
   D Extrapyramidal nervous system.

2. Which one of the following groups contains symptoms which could all be experienced by Gwen in a panic attack?
   A Feelings of guilt, fears of dying and faintness.
   B Blurring of vision, feelings of guilt and fears of dying.
   C Faintness, blurring of vision and feelings of guilt.
   D Fears of dying, faintness and blurring of vision.

3. Which one of the following interventions would be helpful when working with Gwen if she experiences a panic attack?
   A Counselling to talk out fears.
   B Instruction in breathing exercises.
   C Providing a model of calmness and control.
   D Offering physical undemanding tasks.

4. Which one of the following groups contains elements of non-verbal communication which could all be helpful in interactions with Gwen during a panic attack?
   A Stay with her, adopt a non-threatening posture and guide to a chair.
   B Adjust personal space according to client response, stay with her and adopt a non-threatening posture.
   C Guide to a chair, adjust personal space according to client response and stay with her.
   D Adopt a non-threatening posture, guide to a chair and adjust personal space according to client response.

5. Which one of the following groups contains environmental controls which would all be helpful to Gwen whilst she is experiencing severe anxiety?
   A Noise-free, unhurried staff activities and soft furnishings.
   B Unhurried staff activities, soft furnishings and a bright contrasting decor.
   C Soft furnishings, a bright contrasting decor and noise-free.
   D A bright contrasting decor, noise-free and unhurried staff activities.

6. Which one of the following groups contains activities which could all help to reduce Gwen's level of anxiety?
   A Large motor activities, accompanied walks and restrictions on movements.
   B Accompanied walks, restrictions on movements and simple repetitive tasks.
   C Restrictions on movements, simple repetitive tasks and large motor activities.
   D Simple repetitive tasks, large motor activities and accompanied walks.

7. Which one of the following groups contains cognitive tasks which would all help Gwen to manage her levels of anxiety more successfully?
   A Identify trigger factors, understand the relationship between stress and the physical experience of anxiety, and be able to validate reality.
   B Learn alternative coping strategies, identify trigger factors, and understand the relationship between stress and the physical experience of anxiety.
   C Be able to validate reality, learn alternative coping strategies and identify trigger factors.
   D Understand the relationship between stress and the physical experience of anxiety, be able to validate reality and learn alternative coping strategies.

8. Which one of the following groups contains factors which may all form part of a desensitisation programme offered to Gwen?
   A Learn techniques of relaxation, relieve emotions through talking and form a hierachy of anxiety-provoking situations.
   B Be gradually exposed to identified situations, learn techniques of relaxation and relieve emotions through talking.
   C Form a hierachy of anxiety-provoking situations, be gradually exposed to identified situations and learn techniques of relaxation.
   D Relieve emotions through talking, form a hierachy of anxiety-provoking situations and be gradually exposed to identified situations.

9. Which one of the following groups contains elements which could all be offered
   as part of relaxation therapy?
   A Deep muscle relaxation, fantasy and controlled breathing.
   B Passive limb exercises, deep muscle relaxation and fantasy.
   C Controlled breathing, passive limb exercises and deep muscle relaxation.
   D Fantasy, controlled breathing and passive limb exercises.

Answer keys to MCQs

1. The physiological response to anxiety is a complex one involving many systems. The physical response is, however, largely stimulated by sympathetic overactivity of the autonomic nervous system and by the consequent release of adrenalin.

   Option A is the correct response.

   Option B: The pyramidal system is that which forms the tracts between cortex and spinal cord and is concerned with the initiation of movement.

   Option C: The parasympathetic nervous system acts in conjunction with the sympathetic but provides an opposite response.

   Option D: The extrapyramidal system is concerned with the coordination of movement and the provision of fine control.

2. Clients in panic experience many emotional and physical symptoms.

   Option D is the correct response. All the symptoms are associated with panic attacks.
   Feelings of impending doom are common and are likely to be stated as fears of dying, collapse, fainting or loss of control. Somatic symptoms are experienced and include blurring of vision, shortness of breath and palpitations.

   Options A, B and C: All include feelings of guilt. The person in panic is too preoccupied and distressed to give any thoughts to behaviours and their consequences.

3. People in panic are unlikely to have sufficient attention to respond to any teachings, instructions or activities. Interventions should be based on this principle.

   Option C is the correct response. Nursing interventions in panic should be centred on retaining a presence which models calmness and control and offers physical security.

   Option A: Counselling to explore trigger factors and cathartic interventions to facilitate the expression of strong emotions may prove fruitful at times other than panic.

   Option B: Breathing control exercises as a way of reducing anxiety are useful. Instructions in techniques cannot be received by clients in panic.

   Option D: Physical undemanding tasks, especially those which require large motor movements, may be useful in the reduction of anxiety. The client in panic will have insufficient control to engage in such activities.

4. The nurse's use of non-verbal communication provides the best type of intervention for clients in panic. The reasons behind this are: firstly, non-verbal communication is fundamental and directly engages basic needs for security and safety predominant among people experiencing panic; secondly, the degree of attention is so narrowed in acute panic that the content of speech becomes missed.

Option B is the correct response. All the elements indicated would prove helpful. The nurse should stay with the client to provide safety and security as people in panic may put themselves at physical risk. She should adopt an open, non-threatening posture, modelling behaviour which reflects control and calmness. The client's need for personal space should be judged and proximity adjusted according to response. Some clients will find closeness and touch reassuring whilst others may find it intrusive and threatening. In a similar way, some clients will have a need for privacy whilst others will require large open spaces.

Options A, C and D: All include guiding to a chair which may be useful for a limited number of clients but cannot form the basis of an intervention.

5. Control of the environment may help in containing anxiety and should aim to provide a restful unstimulating situation.

Option A is the correct response. All of the stated factors could be helpful. Clients experiencing severe anxiety are hypersensitive to noise and a quiet subdued environment is desirable. Staff rush and bustle should be reduced as such activity can increase environmental stress. Soft furnishings can help to structure the situation towards relaxation.

Options B, C and D: All include a bright contrasting decor which may be cheerful but will tend to increase stimulation and thereby anxiety levels, or at least, make it more difficult to achieve relaxation.

6. A number of activities have been found to help people reduce their levels of anxiety.

Option D is the correct response. All of the stated activities may prove helpful. The provision of simple, repetitive tasks help to divert attention away from negative thoughts. The tasks should not require hard concentration or decision-making. The repetitive nature of a task offers a behaviour without threat or over-stimulation. Large motor activities such as sweeping the floor, digging or making beds help to reduce the physical experience of anxiety by using up free adrenalin. Accompanied walks offer relatedness without threat and the opportunity to talk if this is wanted, rather than an expectation of communication.

Options A, B and C: All include restriction on movement which can feel constraining and mobilise bodily systems rather than calm them.

7. The development of understanding about anxiety and its control can help clients to apply the skills of anxiety management more effectively.

Option B is the correct response. All of the principles stated would be helpful. The learning of alternative coping strategies for anxiety-provoking situations will help clients to respond in ways other than disabling anxiety. The identification of trigger factors may help people to restructure part of their behaviour patterns or at least prepare them for those situations which trigger off anxiety. An understanding of the relationship between stress and the physical symptoms of anxiety will do much to break the feedback loop where physical symptoms act as stressors, creating an escalation of anxiety.

Options A, C and D: All include the validation of reality which is more appropriate to people who confuse or misinterpret reality as in confusion or disorders of thought and perception.

8. Desensitisation is a technique derived from behaviour therapy, based on a process of reciprocal inhibition, where the response of anxiety is replaced by control.

Option C is the correct response. All of the stated activities may form part of a desensitisation programme. One of the first steps in such a programme is to identify anxiety-provoking situations and grade them by response into a hierachy. The learning of relaxation techniques enables the client to link relaxation to those anxiety-provoking situations. This should be done by gradual exposure using simulation, fantasy or real life situations.

Options A, B and D: All include the relief of emotions through talking. This is recognised as useful in the reduction of experienced anxiety but does not form an essential part of a desensitisation programme.

9. There are numerous ways of teaching relaxation therapy but most have certain elements in common.

Option A is the correct response. All of the stated activities are commonly offered. Deep muscle relaxation can be achieved by the alternate contraction and relaxation of muscle groups. The client learns to recognise the symptoms of tension and achieve muscular relaxation which can then be used outside of the sessions. Fantasy may involve the evocation of restful places or the putting aside of anxiety and its substitution by control. Techniques of controlled breathing can also be learned within sessions and applied in situations where anxiety is experienced.

Options B, C and D: All include techniques of massage which can help to induce relaxation but are not under client control. Passive limb exercises are more appropriate as a physical intervention for people whose movements are restricted.

Essay questions

1. Gwen Seymour is a married woman of 35 with two children, a daughter of 13 and a son of 11. She has an irrational fear of leaving the home and now experiences attacks of severe panic if the need to leave the house arises.

   A Describe behaviour that could be observed during an acute panic attack.   20%

   B How should the nurse intervene in order to assist Mrs Seymour in a panic attack?   40%

   C Outline a behaviour therapy programme which the community psychiatric nurse could implement in order to help Mrs Seymour manage her anxiety.   40%

2. Gwen Seymour, aged 35, is married with two children, a girl of 13 and a boy of 11. She is referred to the community psychiatric nursing services because of excessive anxiety upon leaving home.

   A Describe the relationship between stress and the physical experience of anxiety.   20%

   B Describe base-line observations that the community nurse could make of Mrs Seymour and her behaviour.   30%

   C Describe a progressive programme of care which the community psychiatric nurse could implement to help Mrs Seymour with her difficulties.   50%

3. Gwen Seymour, a 35-year-old married woman with two children, a daughter aged 13 and a boy of 11, is referred to the community psychiatric nursing services. Over the last few years she has become increasingly anxious about leaving the home and is now virtually housebound. Her husband John is finding it difficult to maintain the household and remain in employment.

   A Discuss the psychological motives which may have led to the present situation.   20%

   B Describe nursing interventions which could help to reduce anxiety.   50%

   C Discuss the possible effects of this behaviour on the family.   30%

Specimen answer (Essay question 1)

1. A The behaviour that may be observed is that of complete distress. There may
     be an increased psychomotor activity with wild purposeless movements and
     screaming and shouting. Some clients may be rigid and motionless and
     appear frozen and unable to speak. Physical signs of extreme anxiety may be
     present and include sweating, dilated pupils, hyperventilation and trembling.
     The person will not respond to requests or interactions and may complain of
     severe distress, fears of dying and feelings of impending collapse.

   B The nurse should maintain a presence during the attack and safeguard the
     patient from physical harm. She should be aware of her body language which
     should model calmness, control and efficiency. The need for personal space
     should be considered and altered according to client response to proximity or
     touch.

     Verbal interactions should be kept short and be concerned with safety and
     control. The voice should be calm, soft and unhurried and the timing of the
     interactions should coincide with the client's pattern of speech or silence.
     The environment could be controlled so as to reduce stimuli and maintain
     privacy and dignity. Mrs Seymour should be encouraged to use any existing
     anxiety-controlling skills.

   C A behaviour-therapy programme should start with a behavioural analysis
     based on the antecedents, behaviour, consequences model. The antecedents
     would include any trigger factors or situations stimulating anxiety. The
     behaviour could be noted in terms of timing, frequency, length and depth, or
     response. This could be ascertained by observations of the nurse using
     limited exposure techniques, or by the husband, or by self-rating. The
     consequences of the behaviour and response of others in the situation should
     also be assessed.

     Education regarding the nature of stress and the physical experience of
     anxiety could then be offered and involvement of the husband could
     continue. Alternative coping behaviours could be explored. The formulation of
     a hierachy of stress-inducing situations could now be undertaken and involve
     the client, the family and the nurse.

     Anxiety-reduction techniques, such as muscle relaxation and breathing
     control exercises, alongside self-enhancing statements, could be learnt.

     The situations could then be introduced through gradual exposure, linking
     the situation with control and relaxation. These could be worked through by
     simulation, in imagination or in real life. The possibility of regression in
     therapy should be allowed for, the nurse maintaining an optimistic outlook.

     The husband and family need to be aware of the programme and their
     contribution to its success, particularly in redefining roles and responsibilities.

     There should be a gradual relinquishing of support to the client and family.

Answer guides

2. A The relationship between stress and the physical experience of anxiety involves an interplay and feedback between psychological components and physiological responses and may be illustrated by the following flow diagram.

Stress (isolation, insecurity)

↓

Psychological symptoms (fear, apprehension)

↓

Physiological response   autonomic response,
endocrine stimulation

↓   release of adrenalin

Physical symptoms (muscular tension, palpitations)

↓

Increased stress

B Base-line observations could be made on:
— antecedents: where, when, who with
— behaviour: how long, frequency, response
— consequences: reactions of others, changes to situation.

C A progressive programme could include:
— Relationship formation: trust, acceptance, warmth.
— Assessment of problems:
    behavioural analysis
    interviews with client and family
    assessment by other disciplines.
— Interventions:
    education
    behaviour therapy.
— CPN offering support, encouragement, counselling. Assisting the family to redefine roles and responsibilities. Gradual withdrawal of support and giving of responsibility to client and family.
— Evaluation at all stages of the programme in order to adjust the rate of progression to the responses of the client.

3. A Learning theory explanations where the relief of anxiety associated with withdrawal from stimuli acts as the reinforcer for further withdrawal:
— Psychodynamic where the phobic symptoms form the expression of unresolved conflicts.
— Interactionist/life transitions, the interplay of inter- and intrapersonal dynamics.
— Transactional analysis: playing of psychological games as a way of structuring time and accumulating strokes.

B Control of the environment: quiet and restful. Nursing approach to be non-threatening and initially low profile but supportive.
   — Provide relatedness without threat, e.g., accompanied walks.
   — Emotional release through talking and cathartic interventions.
   — Identification of alternative coping strategies.
   — Teaching of anxiety-reduction techniques.
C Effects on husband: frustration, resentment, anger, guilt.
   Effects on children: restriction of opportunities, learned anxieties.
   Family dynamics: deterioration of relationships, reversal of roles and responsibilities.

3. Obsessional ideas and compulsive behaviour as a disturbed coping pattern

Julie Hudson is 25 years old, single and lives at home with her parents. She has no brothers or sisters. According to her parents she has always been a quiet and sensitive girl who has given no cause for concern.

On leaving school she went to work in a local bank where she was well liked by her colleagues. Her appearance is smart; she is fastidious about tidiness and in her private life becomes irritated and upset by any lack of order.

Julie's employers reported that initially they were pleased with her conscientious behaviour. Over the past 2 years, however, she has had to be counselled about delaying the workings of the organisation. Two months ago the bank reluctantly suspended Julie because she had started wearing gloves at work and washing her hands repeatedly between each transaction. Since that time she has begun to experience intrusive thoughts, often of a sexual nature. These thoughts worry and embarrass her. She recognises that they are her own thoughts but no matter how hard she tries she cannot stop them entering her mind.

Although nothing has happened yet, she is constantly afraid that she will embarrass both herself and her family in public.

She has recently been referred to the community psychiatric nursing services by her general practitioner.

Multiple choice questions

1. Which one of the following is most characteristic of an obsessional disorder? That the client:
   A is aware of her thoughts but is unconcerned by them.
   B recognises the irrationality of her thoughts but is unable to control them.
   C is likely to actually carry out the theme of her obsessional thinking.
   D is aware of her thoughts but is convinced that they are being implanted into her mind.

2. Which one of the following groups of symptoms is most likely to be experienced by a person suffering from an obsessional disorder?
   A Ritualistic thoughts, ideas of thought control and feelings of compulsion.
   B Ideas of thought control, feelings of compulsion and feelings of anxiety.
   C Feelings of compulsion, feelings of anxiety and ritualistic thoughts.
   D Feelings of anxiety, ritualistic thoughts and ideas of thought control.

3. Which one of the following groups contains theories which have all been associated with the development of obsessional disorders?
   A Double-bind situations, emotional stress and unresolved conflicts.
   B Emotional stress, unresolved conflicts and early imprinting/socialisation.
   C Unresolved conflicts, early imprinting/socialisation and double-bind situations.
   D Early imprinting/socialisation, double-bind situations and emotional stress.

4. Which one of the following is the most likely explanation for people carrying out compulsive acts? That the acts:
   A allow the external expression of fantasies.
   B prevent or reduce anxiety or tension.
   C are used as a means of gaining attention.
   D enable the individual to develop self-control.

5. Which one of the following groups of nursing skills would be most appropriate when caring for Julie?
   A Offer support, demonstrate acceptance and employ challenging
   B Demonstrate acceptance, employ challenging and encourage exploration.
   C Employ challenging, encourage exploration and offer support.
   D Encourage exploration, offer support and demonstrate acceptance.

6. Which one of the following nursing approaches would be most helpful in assisting Julie to develop control of her behaviour?
   A Discontinue interactions when Julie displays inappropriate behaviour.
   B Give short, repetitive instructions regarding her behaviour.
   C Encourage focussing on problems and the relationship between the problems and anxiety.
   D Suggest that she strives to control behaviours which are unproductive.

7. Which one of the following groups of therapies would be useful in modifying Julie's behaviour?
   A Thought stopping, imagery flooding and in vivo flooding.
   B Imagery flooding, in vivo flooding and aversion therapy.
   C In vivo flooding, aversion therapy and thought stopping.
   D Aversion therapy, thought stopping and imagery flooding.

8. Which one of the following most clearly defines the meaning of reciprocal inhibition? When:
   A the feeling of anxiety is increased when confronted with an appropriate stimulus.
   B an individual attempts voluntarily to limit his or her own behaviour, resulting in a consequent reduction of anxiety.
   C an individual experiences a planned feeling of relaxation under circumstances which normally produce anxiety.
   D a feeling of relaxation is replaced by anxiety through repeated exposure to threatening situations.

9. Which one of the following groups of drugs is most likely to be prescribed for Julie?
   A Anti-depressants.
   B Anxiolytics.
   C Cerebral stimulants.
   D Cortical depressants.

Answer keys to MCQs

1. In obsessional disorders contact with reality is maintained. The client is aware that the thoughts she is experiencing and the behaviours she is exhibiting are inappropriate. Despite this knowledge the person feels unable to control the intrusive or compelling ideas.

   Option B is the correct response.

   Option A   is more like 'la belle indifference' which may be witnessed in individuals displaying conversion symptoms. In obsessional disorders the individual involved is extremely concerned by her thoughts and behaviours.

   Option C   is incorrect as even though the thoughts are demanding and intrusive, very few people put these thoughts into practice. It has been suggested that people who carry out their fantasies in the real world are more likely to be experiencing some form of psychopathic or sociopathic disorder.

   Option D   concerns the belief that thoughts are being implanted in the brain. This is associated with a loss of contact with reality. It is a phenomenon normally included in the general area of ideas of passivity, and as such is more likely to occur in psychotic disorders.

2. A person who experiences obsessional disorders usually maintains her contact with reality, and is aware that something is wrong with her thinking and behaviour.

   Option C is the correct response. The person concerned experiences ritualistic thinking and a feeling of compulsion to do or say things which she realises are inappropriate. The awareness that these symptoms are inappropriate causes a great deal of anxiety.

   Options A, B and D: All include ideas of thought control. This is more likely to be experienced by people who have lost contact with reality. The person who has obsessional ideas knows that they are irrational but is aware that they emanate from her own mind as opposed to being implanted against her will.

3. A number of theories have been proposed regarding the aetiology of obsessional disorders. As with most psychiatric disorders, however, the specific cause remains obscure.

   Option B is the correct response. These are the common psycho-social theories associated with an obsessional disorder. Imprinting and early socialisation relate to patterns of behaviour which are developed during formative periods in an individual's early life. Unresolved conflicts may produce feelings of intense guilt and remorse which may in turn stimulate the development of compensatory or substitutional behaviours. It is also thought that emotional conflict may in some cases precipitate the development of an obsessional disorder.

Options A, C and D: All include double-bind situations. Such conflicts have been associated with the development of other disorders, notably the schizophrenias. The double-bind theory was suggested by Bateson and was concerned with conflict engendered by a discrepancy between what is actually said by significant others, and that which is implied by such things as tone of voice or facial expression.

4. Obsessional behaviours may occur through processes of repression, displacement and substitution. The acts are likely to be associated with feelings of compulsion. The individual will experience a sense of tension if the behaviour is prevented or inhibited.

   Option B is the correct response. Whilst the person concerned feels self-conscious and embarrassed, the subsitutional behaviour may inhibit the development, or produce a reduction in, levels of anxiety.

   Option A: Compulsive acts are not normally a result of fantasies. When such behaviour occurs as an expression of fantasies, it is usually associated with people who have either lost contact with reality, e.g., the schizophrenias, or in individuals who have difficulties in learning and interpersonal relationships, e.g., psychopathic disorders.

   Option C: The person who exhibits this type of behaviour will undoubtedly attract a great deal of attention: the attention, however, will be a consequence of rather than a cause of the behaviour.

   Option D: This is something which in her own way the person would like to achieve. As such it is a desirable outcome of therapy but is not a reason for the behaviour occurring.

5. Julie will, of course, be aware of her behaviours but is likely to feel lost and uncertain as to why she is thinking and behaving as she is. It is possible that in her social contacts she has experienced some ridicule and advice on stopping her behaviour. Embarrassment and feelings of guilt may have occurred as a consequence of these interactions. When therapy starts she may feel uncertain and apprehensive about what is expected of her, and of her own abilities.

   Option D is the correct response. The nurse must demonstrate a sense of acceptance and understanding, that her behaviour is not seen as ridiculous, but as something which she wishes to control but cannot.
   Skills of exploration will be used to help Julie examine her behaviours and the possible relationship between anxiety and the

behaviour. Whilst Julie is progressing through therapy and trying out new behaviours and attempting to establish control, she will require a great deal of support and encouragement.

Options A, B and C: All include the skill of challenging which can be useful in a variety of situations. It is not likely, however, to be of much benefit in helping Julie with her problems.

6. In attempting to help Julie overcome her problems the nurse must adopt an approach which acknowledges and encourages Julie's responsibility for her own care.

   Option C is the correct response. The nurse should help the client to explore and examine the relationship between her problems and anxiety.

   Option A: A response of this type may be appropriate when interacting with a client who displays attention-seeking behaviour. It is not Julie's intention to gain attention through her particular responses to anxiety.

   Option B: This type of interaction would not be of assistance to Julie. The nurse is being directive which removes responsibility for care from Julie. It is the type of response which could be appropriate when caring for a person who was excited or confused.

   Option D: would not provide any assistance to the client. She is already aware that her behaviour is irrational and it is likely that she is already trying hard to exert control.

7. The therapies which appear to be most successful in helping someone with an obsessional disorder are generally behavioural in nature. These are usually concerned with re-learning appropriate, or interrupting inappropriate behaviours.

   Option A is the correct response. Thought stopping is a technique of interrupting the client's thought pattern, commonly verbally. As therapy progresses the client would be encouraged to interrupt her own thoughts at a progressively earlier stage.
   Flooding or implosion therapy is a technique of exposing the client to her worst fears. It is essential that during such therapy the client is provided with much support. The process of flooding may be undertaken using imagery or in vivo (real-life) situations.

   Options B, C and D: All include aversion therapy. Although this is an example of a behaviourist form of therapy, it would not be appropriate for a client experiencing an obsessional disorder.

8. The processes of de-conditioning and covert reinforcement have been shown to have a place in the care of individuals with obsessional disorders. Both utilise the principle of reciprocal inhibition.

Option C is the correct response. This process is aided by the development of relaxation techniques. An alternative is to use a planned reinforcer such as an agreed pleasant thought, as part of covert reinforcement.

Options A, B and C: All include some method of either decreasing or increasing levels of anxiety. None of these embodies the principles of reciprocal inhibition.

9. Obtaining some form of behavioural control involving personal responsibility is most likely to produce benefits which are longer lasting. Other techniques have been suggested, and some, such as the use of medications, are regularly employed. Where chemotherapy is utilised the aim is to interfere with the anxiety-response mechanism physiologically, thereby reducing levels of anxiety.

Option B is therefore the correct response.

Option A: Anti-depressants may at some time be offered in Julie's care, especially if her problems were not resolved and a depressive disorder ensued. They would be of no value in helping Julie with her obsessional behaviour.

Option C would be inappropriate. This type of drug would produce an increase in activity, both cerebral and motor.

Option D: Cortical depressants are preparations which reduce the level of activity within the cerebral cortex. Commonly-used medications which fall within this category are anti-convulsants.

Essay questions

1. Julie is a young woman who lives with her parents; she has recently been referred to the community psychiatric nursing services.

   For the past 2 years she has been troubled by compulsive hand washing, and more recently by feeling the need to wear gloves whilst carrying out her work as a counter assistant in a bank. She was suspended from her job 2 months ago, and since that time thoughts of a sexual nature have repeatedly intruded into her thinking.

   A Discuss the possible psychological motives of obsessional compulsive disorders.   20%

   B Outline the ways in which the nurse may assist Julie to gain control of her behaviour and thoughts.   80%

2. Julie Hudson is 25 years old, single, and lives with her parents.

   She has recently been referred to the community psychiatric nursing services for help with an obsessional compulsive disorder related to cleanliness and intrusive thoughts. These problems resulted in her being suspended from her job as a bank counter assistant 2 months ago.

   A Outline the behavioural techniques which the community nurse may employ to help Julie regain control of her disruptive thoughts and behaviours.   70%

   B How should the nurse respond, giving rationales for the response, when Julie says, 'How am I going to face my friends and workmates after this?'   30%

3. Julie is an only child, single, and lives at home with her parents. They remember her during her developing years as a quiet, shy, and sensitive girl. Two years ago she began to be troubled by thoughts of cleanliness, which subsequently affected her work, resulting in her suspension from employment. Since that time she has also experienced thoughts of a sexual nature. Following consultations with her general practitioner and a psychiatrist, she has been referred to the community psychiatric nursing services.

   A How can the community nurse help Julie's parents when they express concern about the development of these problems, and enquire about ways in which they can best help their daughter?   50%

   B Describe ways in which the nursing staff could help Julie to return to full employment.   50%

Specimen answer

1. A   It is believed that the seeds of obsessional compulsive behaviour are ideas which the individual finds intolerable. These unresolved difficulties produce feelings of great anxiety, guilt and remorse. Because acceptance and externalisation of these ideas would prove so difficult, a process of repression and displacement occurs, producing an apparently unconnected but substitutional behaviour.

 This behaviour, although accepted by the individual as irrational, results in a reduction of his feelings of tension.

   B   The approach of the nurse should be one of acceptance and understanding. Julie may have been ridiculed or chastised by those around her; in addition to which she may, herself, believe that she is 'going mad'.

 The nurse must be prepared to listen to Julie and offer support by being approachable, positive and open in their relationship.

 Julie's involvement in her own care should be promoted from the outset. An early discussion should be instituted to establish antecedents and baseline behaviours. Identification of goals and establishment of care plans must all involve her, and it may be appropriate to consider the use of contractual agreements in the planning of care.

 An examination and exploration of feelings of anxiety and guilt may be undertaken. Care must be taken in this area, for the anxiety and substitutional behaviour may be a protective mechanism which if removed could produce alternative forms of defence.

 The use of behavioural techniques has been found to produce benefits in many people suffering from obsessional compulsive disorders. The nurse should consider techniques such as thought stopping, flooding, covert reinforcement and desensitisation, and be prepared to employ whichever seems most suitable for Julie.

 Diversional techniques may also be utilised. These should not include a great deal of detailed work but could include activities in which Julie has previously experienced enjoyment or success.

 In an attempt to improve Julie's confidence the nurse should give praise where appropriate and in a way which is not condescending. Julie should be encouraged to recognise and acknowledge any achievement, no matter how small. Involvement in new activities can be satisfying in this respect.

 Julie will need a great deal of support throughout the process of behavioural analysis. Help and evaluation can be offered by the nurse; in addition she could be encouraged to attend a non-analytic support group on an out-patient basis.

 The use of medications to help Julie may be minimal; nevertheless the nurse must encourage her to take prescribed medication at the appropriate time.

Answer guides

2. A Behavioural analysis should be the first stage, and would include an examination of antecedents, behaviour and consequences.
    Thought stopping:
    — agreement that thoughts are futile
    — Julie thinks about agreed subject
    — therapist shouts 'Stop!'
    — therapist acknowledges with Julie that thoughts do stop
    — the exercise is repeated several times
    — Julie encouraged to say 'Stop' herself, at a subvocal level
    — client then encouraged to interrupt own thoughts in this way each time
        they return
    — when thought stops, quickly concentrate on something else.
    De-sensitisation:
    — the inhibition of behaviours by a gradual introduction to the source of
        discomfort whilst remaining relaxed.
    Implosion (flooding or response prevention):
        Imagery:
        — under controlled situations Julie would be encouraged to repeatedly
            picture herself in the worst possible situations related to her thoughts
            and behaviours.
        Graduated in-vivo exposure:
        — Julie would be asked to make a list of articles she did not wish to touch.
        — the nurse would then model appropriate responses
        — the client would then touch, in order, the articles of her dislike
        — no washing is allowed for a period of 2 hours
        — repeated exposure can produce a reduction in anxiety and disruptive
            behaviours.
    Covert reinforcement:
    — the client is encouraged to establish a 'reinforcer'
    — under controlled situations Julie is allowed free thought
    — when an obsessional idea occurs Julie signals to the therapist
    — therapist shouts reinforcer
    — Julie then thinks about agreed pleasant situation.
    Objectives group:
    — this is not a form of true behaviour therapy but may help in behavioural
        control
    — group meets weekly
    — each individual identifies achievable goal
    — through the following week, clients attempt to achieve agreed goals
    — at next meeting, discuss the preceding week, offer support and establish
        new goal.
    B Recognise feelings such as embarrassment, guilt or anxiety. Encourage
    ventilation by allowing time, listening and using responding skills.

Offer support using verbal and non-verbal techniques.
Examine strategies to help Julie to confront the problem:
— personal development
— imagination of events
— use of close friends and colleagues.

3. A Approach:
— understand and accept their feelings of guilt, anger, frustration and anxiety.
Offer support.
Examine:
— concerns of parents
— their knowledge base.
Education:
— related to symptoms and Julie's inability to control them.
Encouragement:
— to ventilate feelings
— in their endeavours to understand and help.
Explore ways of helping:
— their part in behavioural techniques
— Julie's need for support and understanding
— the need for regularity in taking medications.
  B The following areas should be considered:
— establish base-line behaviours
— undertake behavioural analysis
— establish goals
— construct a care plan
— involve Julie in all aspects of care
— consider the use of contracts
— style of nursing approach
— details of behavioural interventions
— discuss contacting employer
— provide graded support regarding Julie's return to the work situation
— ensure relevant information is given to Julie's parents.

4. Over-emotional and attention-seeking behaviour as a disturbed coping pattern

Angela Duncan is 22 years old, single and the daughter of parents who are now in their 60s. She experienced problems at school in her relationships with other children and was often kept at home by her mother, who would frequently visit the school in order to complain about the other children and ask for protection for her daughter.

In her adolescence Angela became increasingly emotional and behaved in a distressed manner when difficulties arose. At this time she started hyperventilating which sometimes led to collapse. Later the collapse was accompanied by convulsions and these reactions still persist. Full physical investigations have failed to elicit any organic problem and the cause is now thought to be psychogenic.

She has a lowered self-esteem and feels incapable of leading an independent life-style. In the recent past, when stressful circumstances have become unbearable, she has resorted to acts of deliberate self-harm by attempting to cut her wrists. After the last occasion she was admitted to an acute psychiatric ward.

Her parents visit frequently and engage the nursing staff in lengthy discussions about their daughter's illness and difficulties. On the ward she is described as over-emotional and attention-seeking. She has difficulty in relating to people at anything other than a superficial level.

Multiple choice questions

1. Which one of the following offers the best definition of conversion reactions? That the person experiences:
   A physical changes of psychogenic origin.
   B physical changes of organic origin.
   C physical symptoms of psychogenic origin.
   D physical symptoms of organic origin.

2. Which one of the following groups contains diagnostic criteria which would all suggest a conversion reaction rather than a physical illness?
   A Absence of positive neurological signs, symptoms associated with interpersonal difficulties and failure to respond to usual treatments.
   B Symptoms associated with interpersonal difficulties, failure to respond to usual treatments and concern over symptoms.
   C Failure to respond to usual treatments, concern over symptoms and absence of positive neurological signs.
   D Concern over symptoms, absence of positive neurological signs and symptoms associated with interpersonal difficulties.

3. Which one of the following best describes the concept of primary gain in the development of hysterical behaviour? That the behaviour:
   A reduces intrapersonal anxiety or conflict.
   B is increased by attention from others.
   C is rewarded and thereby reinforced.
   D is initially concerned with gaining sympathy.

4. Which one of the following best describes the concept of secondary gain?
   A The psychological benefits that the client experiences as a result of the symptoms.
   B The benefits accruing to others, arising from the client's symptoms.
   C The reduction of anxiety associated with the development of symptoms.
   D The increase in severity of symptoms over time.

5. Which one of the following groups contains interventions which would all be useful in working with Angela when she responds in dramatic and over-emotional ways?
   A Help the client to identify needs which the behaviour fulfils, take responsibility for determining the range of acceptable behaviour, and discuss and identify alternative ways of behaving.
   B Help client to recognise the consequences of the behaviour, help the client to identify needs which the behaviour fulfils and take responsibility for determining the range of acceptable behaviour.
   C Discuss and identify alternative ways of behaving, help the client to recognise the consequences of the behaviour and help the client to identify needs which the behaviour fulfils.
   D Take responsibility for determining the range of acceptable behaviour, discuss and identify alternative ways of behaving and help the client to recognise the consequences of the behaviour.

6. Which one of the following groups contains nursing interventions which would all be helpful in working with Angela when she adopts attention-seeking behaviour?
   A Encourage the expression of feelings, confront attention-seeking behaviours and ignore the client when the behaviour is maladaptive.
   B Model appropriate ways of communicating needs, encourage the expression of feelings and confront attention-seeking behaviours.
   C Ignore the client when the behaviour is maladaptive, model appropriate ways of communicating needs and encourage the expression of feelings.
   D Confront attention-seeking behaviours, ignore the client when the behaviour is maladaptive and model appropriate ways of communicating needs.

7. Which one of the following groups contains interventions which could all assist Angela to develop more meaningful interpersonal relationships?
   A Give of self in a way which is not dependent upon Angela's demands, use appropriate self-disclosure as a modelling technique and reward constructive, open, social interaction.
   B Use appropriate self-disclosure as a modelling technique, reward constructive, open, social interaction and retain an emotional distance to avoid client manipulation.
   C Reward constructive, open, social interaction, retain an emotional distance to avoid client manipulation and give of self in a way which is not dependent upon Angela's demands.
   D Retain an emotional distance to avoid client manipulation, give of self in a way which is not dependent upon Angela's demands and use appropriate self-disclosure as a modelling technique.

8. Which one of the following groups contains interventions which would all help Angela to build up self-esteem?
   A Provide a schema of success, engage in simple repetitive tasks and involve in activities that give pleasure.
   B Engage in simple repetitive tasks, involve in activities that give pleasure and give of self in a consistent manner.
   C Involve in activities that give pleasure, give of self in a consistent manner and provide a schema of success.
   D Give of self in a consistent manner, provide a schema of success and engage in simple, repetitive tasks.

9. Which one of the following groups contains factors which would all indicate that the lethality risk associated with Angela's behaviour was low?
   A Acts of self-harm related to family disagreements, many previous acts of self-harm and acts of self-harm carried out whilst alone.
   B Acts of self-harm as a way of manipulating others, acts of self-harm related to family disagreements and many previous acts of self-harm.
   C Acts of self-harm carried out whilst alone, acts of self-harm as a way of manipulating others and acts of self-harm related to family disagreements.
   D Many previous acts of self-harm, acts of self-harm as a way of manipulating others and acts of self-harm carried out whilst alone.

Answer keys to MCQs

1. A conversion reaction is one in which psychological conflict is transformed into a physical manifestation.

    Option C   is the correct response. The client complains of various symptoms but no physical cause can be detected.

    Option A   is more akin to psychosomatic disorders where actual physical or organic changes as well as symptoms occur.

    Option B   is a description of true physical disorder.

    Option D   is similarly a description of organic illness.

2. There are a number of ways in which conversion reactions can be differentiated from physical illness. These need to be taken together rather than in isolation, and a full physical investigation is essential before a diagnosis or assessment of hysterical disorder is made.

    Option A   is the correct response: all of the criteria are associated with conversion reactions. There is an absence of positive neurological signs so that the displayed signs and symptoms fail to correspond to that expected. The occurrence is often linked to interpersonal conflicts and difficulties and may well appear convenient. A failure to respond to usual treatments is also likely to be noticed because of the lack of physical pathology.

    Options B, C and D: All contain concern over symptoms. This is in opposition to the usual observation which is of noticeable lack of affect in response to the apparent severity of the symptoms. This is so characteristic that the term 'la belle indifference' has been used to describe it.

3. Primary gain relates to the initial resolution of intrapersonal conflict which the symptoms bring to the client. The process is one of repression, disassociation and displacement.

    Option A   is the correct response. Anxiety is not usually manifest. Instead the anxiety has been displaced and made manifest in the symptoms, bringing psychological relief to the individual.

    Option B   is a reference to secondary gain.

    Option C   is a description of operant conditioning.

    Option D   is more akin to a process in malingering.

4. The conversion reaction usually places the client in the sick role which carries with it a number of nurturing expectations of others. These benefits form the secondary gain which the person derives as a result of illness.

Option A is the correct response.

Option B   places the focus on significant others who may well be colluding with the client for some unresolved needs of their own.

Option C   provides a description more related to the concept of primary gain.

Option D   relates to chronicity which may occur as a result of secondary gain.

5. Clients who respond in over-dramatic ways often do so as a means of gaining sympathy, and may be unaware that their behaviour may give rise to an opposite reaction.

Option C is the correct response. All of the interventions may prove useful. Helping the client understand needs which the behaviour fulfils is one of the first steps in enabling more appropriate ways of asking for needs to be met. A further step is to discuss and identify alternative behaviours which the client may wish to test out. Helping Angela to recognise the consequences of over-emotional behaviour may help her to become aware of the counterproductive effect of her behaviour.

Options A, B and D: All contain interventions which take responsibility for client actions. Angela needs to be involved in all discussions relating to the acceptability and control of different behaviours for any limit-setting programme to achieve success.

6. A number of different nursing interventions may prove useful when working with clients exhibiting attention-seeking behaviours.

Option B is the correct response. All of these interventions may prove useful. The client should be encouraged to express feelings rather than to act them out. The client's behaviour should be confronted in a calm and straightforward manner without paying too much attention to it. If nursing staff can model behaviours of openness and a willingness to express needs and feelings, then the client may be able to learn from them.

Options A, C and D: All include ignoring the client. A better intervention is to minimise the response to maladaptive behaviour and to give attention which is not conditional on client demands.

7. A problem in making other than superficial relationships with people is sometimes found with psychiatric clients. The nurse's ability to give of self in therapeutic ways provides the main principles of intervention.

Option A is the correct response as all of the interventions may prove useful. Giving of self in a way which is not dependent on client demands reinforces the principle of unconditional positive regard without rewarding and encouraging maladaptive and superficial communications. The nurse's ability to use appropriate self-disclosure, especially in respect of needs and feelings, mirrors for the client a model of openness and genuineness. The rewarding of constructive, open, social interaction provides a supportive therapeutic environment in which the client can try out new behaviours and receive appropriate feedback about them.

Options B, C and D: All include retaining an emotional distance which will do nothing for the client's ability to make other than superficial relationships.

8. Clients who adopt demanding and dependent postures often do so from a basis of low self-esteem. A number of styles of intervention may help these individuals to build up a more positive concept of self.

Option C contains interventions which could all prove useful. Involvement in activities that give pleasure do much to build up self-worth. Fun and joy are essential for the maintenance of positive regard for the self in particular and life in general. The giving of self is the most valuable thing that one human being can give to another and confirms the intrinsic value of the other as a worthwhile person. Providing a schema of success and encouraging the client's progress through that may well give opportunities for achievement which have been denied for a long time.

Options A, B and D: All contain engaging in simple repetitive tasks. This may be useful in anxiety or problems of reality testing but will not prove worthwhile in building up a client's self-esteem.

9. Suicidal behaviour should always be taken seriously and given due attention. Certain factors can help to determine the risk of fatality and thereby help the nurse to plan appropriate intervention.

Option B is the correct response. All the factors are associated with a lowered risk. Acts of self-harm associated with manipulating others denote that the main focus of energy is on the playing of psychological games rather than the ending of life. Family disagreements as a motivator are also suspect, though acute crises in relationships may favour a high risk. A number of previous attempts may suggest a low lethality risk, though it must be remembered that a number of people do proceed to suicide after previous attempts.

Options A, C and D: All contain acts of self-harm carried out whilst alone. This carries a higher risk factor as the chances of intervention are lower.

Essay questions

1. Angela Duncan is a 22-year-old single woman, the daughter of doting parents now in their 60s.

   She was admitted to an acute psychiatric ward following self-inflicted superficial cuts to her wrists.

   On the ward, particularly at busy times, she tends to hyperventilate leading to collapse and convulsions. At other times she behaves in over-dramatic and demanding ways, causing difficulties within the ward community.

   A Describe possible attitudes of the nursing staff towards Angela and her behaviour.   25%

   B How could the nursing staff be helped to respond to this over-dramatic and demanding behaviour in an effective way?   50%

   C Describe how Angela's parents may have contributed towards her present behaviour.   25%

2. Angela Duncan is admitted to the ward following an act of deliberate self-harm. She has a history of hyperventilation accompanied by collapse and convulsions. Full physical examination has failed to reveal any disease process and the cause is now thought to be psychogenic.

   On the ward she is described as over-emotional and attention seeking.

   A Describe the process of hyperventilation and its effects.   30%

   B How should nursing staff attempt to meet Angela's needs without reinforcing dependency?   70%

3. Angela Duncan, aged 22, is a patient on an acute psychiatric unit. Her behaviour is described as over-emotional and demanding. At times she tends to hyperventilate and this sometimes leads to collapse and convulsions. No physical illness has been identified.

   A Describe a behavioural analysis that may be undertaken as part of the assessment process.   30%

   B Describe a care programme based upon the results of the behavioural analysis, designed to modify Angela's responses.   70%

Specimen answer

1. A An attitude of non-acceptance of Angela and her behaviour may well develop amongst staff and be expressed towards her. Some members of staff may feel exasperated, with the result that resentment and hostility develop. Such feelings may lead to actions characterised by blaming and scapegoating or criticism and rejection.

   The expression of negative feelings and actions towards Angela may lead to staff feeling guilty and becoming over-solicitous. There is a risk that some staff members actions become inconsistent, with periods of rejection alternating with those of over-protectiveness.

   Other staff may misunderstand the nature of Angela's problems and respond to her emotional and physical problems by over-protectiveness, thus increasing Angela's dependent behaviours.

   A more positive attitude would be one that reflected an acceptance of Angela whilst maintaining an effective stance in regard to her behaviour. The nurse should show an acceptance of Angela which is not dependent on demands or attention-seeking behaviours.

   B It is essential that all staff act in a consistent and enabling way if any change is to be instituted in Angela's behaviour.

   All staff need to be aware of the reasons underlying Angela's behaviour and her likely past experience of reinforcement of maladaptive responses. They need to understand that the behaviour is not consciously motivated but is an expression of underlying unfulfilled needs.

   Nursing staff should be encouraged to examine their own attitudes towards Angela. If these are found to be negative in nature, then assistance should be given to develop attitudes and responses which are more therapeutic. A safe environment in which to air negative feelings should be offered. A system of support and supervision would be helpful for all those who work closely with Angela. Training in interpersonal skills in this area could be offered using exercises, simulations and role play.

   Senior staff on the ward should present effective models of skilled and therapeutic communications.

   C Angela's parents are described as doting and this may well have played a part in the development of her behaviour.

   The parents were in their late 40s when Angela was born and may have lavished inordinate attention upon her and tried to satisfy her every whim. If they were over-anxious about Angela's physical well-being, then a process of over-attention to physical illness could have prevailed.

   Angela could have been given extra attention when sick, thus reinforcing the benefits of showing physical symptoms. Later Angela could have used the development and expression of physical symptoms as a means of deriving secondary gain.

It is possible that the parents maintained their relationship with Angela on an adult-to-child basis, thereby fostering dependency and interfering with the maturational tasks of adolescence.

Answer guides

2. A Hyperventilation:
   — short frequent breaths
   — shallow ventilation
   leads to:
   — disturbance of blood chemistry
   — dizziness, fainting, collapse.
   B Help to identify needs which behaviour fulfils, identify and explore alternative ways of fulfilling needs. Consistent nursing approach:
   — calm, modelling behaviours of control
   — open, showing appropriate expression of feelings
   — confronting, pointing out limits of behaviour
   — accepting of client not necessarily actions
   — challenging, seeking to enable Angela to understand her behaviour
   — supporting, as Angela tries out new ways of relating to others
   — non-defensive, minimal reaction to maladaptive responses
   — encouraging Angela to verbalise rather than act out her feelings.
   Respond to demands without undue attention.
   Consistent response from all staff.
   Evaluate need for assistance and modify as required.

3. A *Behavioural analysis*
   Antecedents:
   — Where does the behaviour occur:
       open, public, private, indoors?
   — Who is there:
       patients, doctors, nurses, parents?
   — What is happening:
       demands on patient, inattention, boredom?
   Behaviour:
   — How many times in a day/hour?
   — How long does it persist?
   — What is the intensity?
   Consequences:
   — What happens then?
   — Who does what?
   — What does patient do/not do?
   B The programme would aim to modify the behaviour by modifying the antecedents, responses or consequences identified in the analysis.

The antecedents could be adjusted, e.g.:
— help the patient to recognise the cues for her behaviour
— alter the environment or the responses of significant people.
The behavioural response could be altered, lessened, e.g.:
— encourage alternative behaviours such as talking
— reward adaptive behaviours.
The consequences could be modified or diminished, e.g.:
— modify the rewards, attention
— restructure the patient's day.

5. Eating disorder as a disturbed coping pattern

Lynne Sweeting is 1.68 m (5 ft 6 in) tall, 24 years old, and has been married to Alistair for 2 years. She has recently been admitted to the female acute ward of a psychiatric unit.

Lynne is one of two children; during her developing years she was somewhat over-protected and led a sheltered life. She appears to have a healthy relationship with her brother who is 4 years her junior. Lynne is described by all the family as being of anxious disposition with a fastidious and orderly approach to life.

When she left school at 18 she found employment as a nanny and appeared to enjoy this work. After 2 years, however, she felt that she wanted a change and took a job as a dental receptionist, a post which she currently holds.

Since the age of 17 Lynne has been concerned about the type of food she eats, preferring whole foods and white meat.

Approximately 3 years ago the family noticed that she was losing weight but did not feel that it was to any significant degree; 1 year ago her parents and Alistair were becoming concerned and persuaded her to see a doctor. Since that time she has continued to lose weight and has undergone numerous physical investigations which have all proved negative. Her general practitioner has referred Lynne to a psychiatrist who has recommended a period of in-patient care.

Following initial interviews and investigations a medical diagnosis of anorexia nervosa was made; her current weight is 39.4 kg (6 st 3 lb).

Multiple choice questions

1. Which one of the following groups contains features which are all commonly seen in people who are suffering from anorexia nervosa?
   A Amenorrhoea, increased activity and lanugo.
   B Increased activity, lanugo and lethargy.
   C Lanugo, lethargy and amenorrhoea.
   D Lethargy, amenorrhoea and increased activity.

2. Which one of the following is the most accurate definition of bulimia nervosa?
   A Ingestion of large quantities of food followed by copious vomiting.
   B Reduction of food intake associated with regular, induced vomiting.
   C Increase in food consumption as a compensatory act.
   D Reduction of food intake resulting in physical and psychological changes.

3. Which one of the following is the most likely reason for Lynne wearing loose-fitting clothing? Because:
   A such clothing does not restrict air flow or circulation, consequently she feels warmer.
   B wearing such garments conceals the extent of her weight loss.
   C this type of clothing is associated with children and wearing it becomes an outward expression of her desire not to grow up.
   D she feels that such clothes are more masculine and thereby serve as a denial of her gender.

4. Which one of the following gives the most appropriate response of the nurse when Lynne throws the food she is offered onto the floor? The nurse should:
   A clean up the food and explain to Lynne that it will be brought back to her later.
   B leave the food on the floor and explain that when she is ready to eat she knows where the food is.
   C sit with Lynne and attempt to discover the reason underlying the action.
   D give the food back where appropriate and state that she will stay until Lynne has eaten it.

5. Which one of the following styles of therapy is most likely to be used in an attempt to help Lynne?
   A Behavioural modification programme.
   B Stimulant drugs.
   C Modified insulin therapy.
   D Electro-convulsive therapy.

6. Which one of the following groups contains factors which would all be important when planning meals for Lynne in the early stages of care? That the food is:
   A rich in protein, rich in carbohydrates and given in small amounts.
   B rich in carbohydrates, given in small amounts and presented frequently.
   C given in small amounts, presented frequently and rich in protein.
   D presented frequently, rich in protein and rich in carbohydrates.

7. Which one of the following is the most likely reason for Lynne's relatives being discouraged from visiting in the initial stages of her care? Because:
   A both parties will find visiting upsetting.
   B visits must be 'earned' as part of Lynne's behavioural programme.
   C it would be a demonstration that the staff have now assumed control of her life.
   D family relationships are the probable cause of Lynne's problems.

8. Which one of the following would be an important element to include in a contract established with Lynne?
   A Her perception of the problem.
   B The perceptions of the family about the problem.
   C Date of discharge.
   D Target weight.

9. Which one of the following medications is most likely to be prescribed for Lynne?
   A Sodium valproate.
   B Insulin.
   C Digoxin.
   D Chlorpromazine.

Answer keys to MCQs

1. There are many features associated with anorexia nervosa. It is generally accepted that for a diagnosis of anorexia nervosa to be made, the client must demonstrate an unwillingness to ingest or retain food. Significant weight loss related to build and age, and a disturbance in menstruation, are other features.

   Other common symptoms are the presence of lanugo, a fine downy hair growth often found on the back, constipation, hypotension, low body temperature and a paradoxical increase in activity.

   Option A is therefore the correct response. All of the features are found in anorexia nervosa.

   Options B, C and D: All include lethargy. As has been noted the opposite of this is usually the case, with the individual displaying seemingly tireless behaviour.

2. Over a number of years a distinction has been made between anorexia nervosa and bulimia nervosa.

   Classically, a client who suffers from anorexia will refrain from eating anything or vomit back normal meals which she has recently ingested.

   In bulimia, however, the client gorges herself on foods, often rich in carbohydrates, to a point where the stomach can no longer cope and regurgitation occurs.

   Option A is the correct response.

   Option B   would be a more appropriate definition for anorexia nervosa.

   Option C   is a description of a substitutional act which occurs in many individuals, often associated with feelings of anxiety.

   Option D   could be an alternative description of anorexia rather than bulimia nervosa.

3. Clients who suffer from anorexia nervosa often display contradictory attitudes towards their weight. There may be statements of a positive nature regarding their weight loss, suggesting the belief that they will, or do look better at this specific weight. At the same time the individual may choose to wear large, loose-fitting clothes designed to hide weight loss from others.

   Option B is the correct response. Usually only the client and her closest relatives appreciate that she has lost weight.

   Option A: Lynne will experience feelings of coldness, even in conditions which others consider comfortable. Whilst some type of clothing can specifically assist in maintaining body temperature, it is not likely that Lynne's choice of clothing is for this reason.

Option C: The client may have an inner desire not to grow up; however the wearing of loose-fitting clothes is not restricted to children.

Option D: This may well be a feeling which she experiences but it is unlikely to be the reason why she chooses to wear such clothes.

4. This type of reaction is one which may well have proved successful in the home environment. In order to defuse a tense situation the family could have agreed to remove the food for the time being. Lynne might now be testing the reactions of those around her to the same behaviours and observing the results. In such circumstances the nurse must remain calm, consistent but firm, and demonstrate to Lynne that her behaviour will not be allowed to achieve the desired aim.

Option D is the correct response. The nurse is showing Lynne that the food must be eaten and that if she throws it away it will be returned to her; she will then be observed until she has eaten.

Option A would only reinforce Lynne's behaviour; she would quickly learn that when her food is thrown to the floor it is taken away from her.

Option B is similar to the response contained in option A; it is, however, more punitive in style and as such is inappropriate.

Option C would be inappropriate as the reasons for her behaviour are already known, to sit with Lynne and explore the reasons would therefore be of little value.

5. A variety of treatment methods have been tried with clients suffering from anorexia nervosa. It would appear that methods which directly change or re-establish eating patterns, associated with subsequent examination of family dynamics, have produced some success.

Option A is the correct response. Some form of behavioural programme based on agreed goals and reward systems should be implemented.

Option B: Stimulant drugs are likely to increase energy and decrease the desire for food which is in direct opposition to the aims of treatment in anorexia nervosa.

Option C has been used in the treatment of anorexia as a means of stimulating appetite. This is inappropriate as appetite is not normally lost.

Option D: Electro-convulsive therapy may be used with clients who are suffering from anorexia nervosa, but only if the client is depressed or the reluctance to eat is threatening life. If the latter is the case such treatment may reduce the resistance of the client to food. Nevertheless it is not a likely form of treatment.

6. In the early stages of care the overriding aim is to re-establish a regular pattern of eating for Lynne. Intake of food by mouth would minimise the necessity of resorting to naso-gastric or parenteral feeding.

   Option B is the correct response. The diet should contain carbohydrates, which are high in calorific value. For Lynne's comfort the meal should be offered in small amounts on a regular basis. The ingestion of large amounts after a period of abstention might produce vomiting or gastro-intestinal disorders. To avoid gastric irritation a bland milky diet could be offered.

   Options A, C and D: All include the concept of a diet which contains a high proportion of protein. This would not be as appropriate as the other choices as the aim is to increase weight in the quickest way possible. Some protein must of course be included in the diet but need not be excessive.

7. A common method of helping people who suffer from anorexia nervosa is to employ a behavioural approach based on rewarding achievement.
   The rewards to be used in such a system must be agreed upon by the client and the therapists. Because of the significance of the family in most relationships, they are often used as part of the reward scheme.

   Option B is therefore the correct response.

   Option A   is probably a correct statement. However, it would not be used as a reason for preventing visiting. It may even be seen as a reason for increasing family involvement.

   Option C: The aim in therapy is to encourage Lynne and the team to work as a unit with shared responsibilities. To achieve this Lynne must be left with as much personal control as possible.

   Option D: Family relationships may indeed be a factor in the development of anorexia nervosa. Individual perceptions and family dynamics must be explored as part of the overall care programme. The possibility of relationships being involved would not alone be sufficient to suggest the withdrawal of visiting rights.

8. For Lynne and the therapists to work towards the same goals on an agreed path, a contract of care may be established. The contract should include details of goals, plans of actions and the nature and format of rewarding.

   Option D is the correct response as it identifies a specific goal. This may be a long-term goal, with those of a more short-term nature being detailed in the care plan.

   Options A and B: Individual perceptions of the problems should be obtained from Lynne and her close relatives. This information would be gathered as part of the initial and ongoing assessment procedure. It should not be included in a contract of care.

Option C   would be inappropriate due to the variables involved in establishing a date of discharge.

9. Chemotherapy may be used to help clients who suffer with anorexia nervosa. Should this be the case, it would usually be as an adjunct to psychologically-based therapies.

Option D is the correct response. Chlorpromazine has been widely used in the treatment of this condition for many years. It is believed that its effectiveness is due to the reduction of anxiety. The reluctance of the client to eat is thereby reduced and weight increase is more likely.

Option A: Sodium valproate is an example of an anti-convulsant drug. As such it would not be used in the treatment of anorexia nervosa.

Option B: Insulin therapy has been used extensively in the treatment of this condition. The main function of this type of treatment is to stimulate appetite. Appetite is not absent in clients who suffer from anorexia nervosa, and as difficulties may arise with clients who are emaciated insulin is now rarely used.

Option C: Digoxin is a drug used to decrease and strengthen the contraction of the heart: it would not be appropriate in the treatment of anorexia nervosa.

Essay questions

1. Lynne is married, 1.68 m (5 ft 6 in) in height and currently weighing 39.4 kg (6 st 3lb). A diagnosis of anorexia nervosa has recently been made.

    She has been seen by her general practitioner and following referral to a psychiatrist, a period of in-patient care has been recommended.

    A Describe a behavioural programme which might be implemented to help this patient.   70%

    B Outline two other forms of therapy which might be considered as a means of helping Lynne.   30%

2. Lynne is a 24-year-old dental receptionist who has recently been admitted to hospital.

    A diagnosis of anorexia nervosa has been made.

    A Outline the factors which are thought to be influential in the development of this condition.   25%

    B Describe the features which would confirm a diagnosis of anorexia nervosa.   25%

    C Describe the qualities and skills which members of the nursing team must display when caring for Lynne.   50%

3. Lynne Sweeting has been married to Alistair for 2 years and works as a dental receptionist.

    Her parents state that during adolescence she was quiet, fastidious and rather anxious. Lynne, however, feels that she was a normal teenager, but was restricted in her activities by her parents, who were concerned about her well-being.

    Over the past 3 years she has gradually lost weight and currently weighs 39.4 kg (6 st 3 lb). After visits from her general practitioner and a psychiatrist she has agreed to a period of in-patient care.

    A How might Lynne's problems have affected the rest of her family?   40%

    B Describe the help which other members of the family might be offered from the nursing services.   60%

Specimen answer

1. A At the start of Lynne's care an initial interview must be conducted. The therapist should use this to develop a relationship between Lynne and the carers based on an atmosphere of 'work'. The inteviews should be with individual family members first, and later with all the family together in order to assess more closely the dynamics of the family unit. The therapist could use this time to show Lynne by word and gesture that she understands her fears. Initially the therapist could suggest to Lynne that she aims to arrest weight loss rather than actually try to gain weight. Conflict situations should be avoided so that an atmosphere of trust can develop.

Associated with the initial interviews, baseline observations of weight and eating patterns will be recorded.

A contract must be established between Lynne and the carers. This should include such aspects as target weight, short-term goals, and rewards to be obtained following achievement of the goals. The reward system must be agreed between both parties and include things which Lynne likes, such as magazines, or are dear to her, such as visits from family or friends. When discussing the care programme with other members of the family, care must be taken to explain Lynne's probable attempts at manipulation. It is common for clients experiencing this condition to ask for items such as laxatives to be brought to them or sent in the mail. Requests of this nature are often accompanied by pleas not to inform or bother the nurses as 'they are too busy' or 'they don't like me'.

At the beginning of the programme Lynne should be confined to bed; this prevents overactivity and assists the carers in maintaining careful observation. Whilst on bed rest she should be asked to use a commode rather than visit the toilet.

A regime of regular eating should be established as quickly as possible. The food concerned has to be to the client's liking and may have to be bland and non-irritating to avoid gastric disturbance. Small amounts should be given regularly to prevent gastric distention and discomfort. The meals should be rich in carbohydrates. When a meal is given to the client the nurse should stay with her and observe that she takes the food. During this time the nurse must project a positive and objective approach, displaying a simple but firm expectation that Lynne will eat. If Lynne responds to the nurse by hurling abuse, or even the food, she should react in a calm manner, removing the food from the floor and obtaining new supplies.

Each day Lynne should be weighed and this weight carefully recorded. The weight check should be at the same time each day, after she has emptied bowels and bladder. The nurse must ensure that the client does not try to artificially increase her weight prior to weighing by consuming large amounts of liquid.

Lynne must be carefully observed as her methods of disposing of food may be quite ingenious. She may for example push biscuits down the backs of pictures or wardrobes, or vomit into plastic bags which she can then throw out of open windows.

In implementing the programme there is a need for nursing staff to be consistent in their approaches and ensure that any rewards earned are given correctly and promptly. At all times a supportive and encouraging attitude must be displayed, perhaps by a positive remark when some small goal is achieved. The nurse should also remember that weight gain may be relatively rapid at first and then slow down.

Great efforts must be made to ensure that Lynne's dignity is maintained as much as possible. This is particularly important when considering the requirements of the programme i.e., bed rest, use of commodes, regular weighing and having to ask for all things.

Throughout the period of care the nurse must display a non-threatening approach. When an attitude of non-acceptance is projected it serves only to damage relationships which have been established, and demonstrates a lack of understanding on the part of the carers.

B A variety of other forms of therapy may be recommended to help Lynne; however, the two most likely are chemotherapy and psychotherapy.

Chlorpromazine has been extensively used in the treatment of anorexia nervosa. It is believed that its mode of action is to reduce levels of anxiety in the sufferer. As the anxiety may be associated with food and eating, a reduction in the anxiety may bring about some improvement in the reluctance of the client to eat.

Psychotherapy is commonly used as an adjunct to behavioural forms of therapy. This is usually commenced after the weight of the client has been increased to an acceptable level. The aim of psychotherapy would be to help Lynne explore the factors which may underlie the development and maintenance of her problems. Strong client–therapist attachments may develop in this situation and it may be advisable to use different therapists for the individual and family work.

Answer guides

2. A *Factors to be considered include*:
Relationship difficulties:
— often between mother and daughter
— over- protectiveness
— domineering
— ambivalence concerning development.
Analytic view:
— fear of becoming pregnant
— association between food and impregnation.
Social influences:
— the 'ideal' woman image

— conflict between slim and 'curvy'
— displacement of anxiety onto food and eating.
Social class:
— most common in classes 1 and 2
— rarely found in classes 4 and 5.
Pre-morbid personality:
— often obsessional, meticulous.
Family illness:
— mother is often suffering physical or emotional illness.
Extension of dieting:
— is possible but uncommon.

B *The classical triad of signs or symptoms associated with anorexia nervosa are*:
Rejection of food.
Loss of weight:
— with no organic cause
— loss of 10% or more from acceptable weight.
Amenorrhoea:
— lasting for 3 months or more.
Other features which may be present are:
— overactivity
— lanugo—growth of fine downy hair, often on the back
— appearance—loose-fitting clothing
— attitude:
    denial of problem
    inability to appreciate what the fuss is about
    usually referred by another family member
— other physical factors:
    constipation
    hypotension
    hypothermia
    dehydration
    bradycardia.

C Relationship development:
— honesty
— openness
— mature respect
— establishing trust.
Assessment skills:
— observation
— interviewing
— data collection.
Planning skills:
— data interpretation
— establishment of priorities

— setting of goals
— establishing contract
— developing care programme
— communication.
Implementation skills:
— behavioural techniques
— reassurance
— persuasion and encouragement
— support
— observation
— counselling, i.e. confronting, challenging
— modelling mature responses.
Evaluation skills:
— observation
— interviewing
— data comparisons.
Qualities:
— consistency
— tact
— understanding
— patience
— firmness
— perseverance.

3. A The disorder of anorexia nervosa is so pervasive that the following feelings in any combination may be experienced by the husband, parents or brother of the client:
— guilt
— anger
— ambivalence
— bewilderment
— impotence—regarding their course of action.
These feelings may lead to the behaviours of:
— withdrawal
— rejection
— disharmony may be created or increased.
In addition to the above, all of the family's energy will be centred upon Lynne and her eating. This preoccupation can lead to the family relinquishing other interests or contacts.

B Understanding of feelings such as guilt, anger, impotence and the associated reactions.
Reassurance regarding progress and future.
Support:
— through psychotherapy

— through care programme
— during period of after-care.
Education:
— of what is meant by anorexia nervosa
— treatment programmes
— sources of help
— their part in care.
Involvement:
— in care programme
— use of contracts
— restriction of visiting.
Psychotherapy:
— establishing the climate
— explanation of purpose
— format of therapy—individual and then group
— encourage:
      examination of relationships
      open discussion
      ventilation of feelings.

6. Reaction to loss

Susan is a 34-year-old patient who has been transferred to a psychiatric ward from a medical ward.

She was brought up in an apparently stable family, the only child of a bank manager and his wife. Both parents are still alive, although her father has recently taken early retirement from his job following medical advice.

When she left school Susan commenced nurse training and ultimately qualified. This is the only work she has ever done.

She had quite a close circle of friends and a satisfactory social life. At 20 she met and started seeing regularly Nick, her first 'real' boyfriend. When she was 22 they agreed to buy and share a home together.

The couple had a daughter when Susan was 26 and it was to look after her that she decided, when pregnant, that she would discontinue working.

According to Susan the current problems started approximately 4 years ago when she wanted to increase their family and Nick disagreed. Since that time the arguments and unpleasantness have gradually increased. However, 3 months ago a crisis point was reached when Nick informed her that he was leaving as he had met someone else. Two weeks after his departure he wrote to her to remind her that the house was in joint names and although it was difficult he now needed his share of the money.

Initially she hid her feelings very well from her family, but in the privacy of her own home she would weep a lot. She regularly telephoned Nick at home and at work, pleading with him to return, promising that she would do anything if only he would come back. When he refused she occasionally made veiled threats to harm herself.

After he had been gone for 2 months the situation became noticeable to others. She was losing interest in herself and her responsibilities, stating that she felt unwanted by anyone. At this time she contacted her family asking them to intervene and speak to Nick. She also asked repeatedly, what she was going to do?

In addition to her general neglect and loss of confidence she was developing feelings of guilt about her inability to satisfy the needs of her daughter at this time.

Exactly 3 months after Nick had left she attempted to take her own life by ingesting 15–20 aspirin tablets.

Multiple choice questions

1. Which one of the following most clearly indicates the stage of loss which Susan was going through when she repeatedly rang Nick?
   A Denial.
   B Bargaining.
   C Anger.
   D Depression.

2. Which one of the following strategies would be the most useful for Susan at the present time? Involvement in:
   A activities which promote the expression of feelings.
   B solo pursuits which afford an opportunity to reflect.
   C activities which serve to help others.
   D pursuits which may be continued later as hobbies.

3. Which one of the following would be the most appropriate response if Susan's parents stated, 'This should never have happened—where have we gone wrong'?
   A 'Don't blame yourselves, she'll be alright.'
   B 'I realise it must be difficult for you, but what could you have done?'
   C 'I can arrange for you to talk to the doctor if you would like.'
   D 'You're obviously upset about Susan, would you like to talk about it some more?'

4. Which one of the following groups of nursing attributes or skills is most likely to engender in Susan feelings of confidence and trust in the nurse?
   A Honesty, acceptance, encouragement and consistency.
   B Acceptance, encouragement, consistency and reliability.
   C Encouragement, consistency, reliability and honesty.
   D Consistency, reliability, honesty and acceptance.

5. Which one of the following indicates the best method for exploring Susan's feelings?
   A Open-ended questions.
   B Empathic approach.
   C Consistent and trustworthy approach.
   D Ensuring time for talking.

6. Which one of the following is the best definition of the responding skill being used if the nurse says to Susan, 'It seems as though you feel lost and uncertain, and this is upsetting you'?
   A Paraphrasing.
   B Clarifying.
   C Reflecting.
   D Summarising.

7. Which one of the following groups of skills would be most appropriate in assisting Susan to develop an independent life?
   A Supporting, encouraging, educating and counselling.
   B Encouraging, educating, counselling and instructing.
   C Educating, counselling, instructing and supporting.
   D Counselling, instructing, supporting and encouraging.

8. Which one of the following interventions would be the most appropriate for the nurse to use if Susan said, 'Why are you always watching me?'?
   A Explain that it is the responsibility of the nurse to observe everyone.
   B Point out that she is concerned about Susan and she does not want her to harm herself again.
   C Apologise, and ensure that any future observation is carried out more discreetly
   D Ask Susan what is making her angry and offer to discuss her feelings with her.

9. Which one of the following indicates the best reason for ensuring that Susan feels supported during therapy?
   A It is essential that she does not feel that she is on her own.
   B It is apparent from her background that she is a woman who requires a lot of support.
   C Without support she may feel it necessary to withdraw from therapy.
   D During therapy interpersonal issues will have to be dealt with and new behaviours tested.

Answer keys to MCQs

1. It may be argued that individuals experience actual or threatened loss through such events as bereavement, termination of a relationship, loss of status or loss of limb. During this process the person may go through the stages of denial, bargaining, anger, depression and ultimately acceptance. These stages cannot of course be separated as compartments in a drawer, but are vague and interwoven.

   Option B is the correct response, exemplified by statements such as: 'If only you will come back I'll do anything.'

   Option A   Denial statements are such as: 'It can't be true, I must have misunderstood.'

   Option C   Anger statements and reactions are such as: 'Why me?' or 'Why my child, husband etc.' when given bad news.

   Option D   Depression can occur and may be recognised by expressions of low self-worth, futility and slowing of physical reactions.

2. Attempted self-harm may be a response to feelings of anger and frustration. As such, forms of activity are required which allow for the expression of the energy associated with these feelings.

   Option A is the correct response.

   Option B   is incorrect because Susan requires contact with others to develop her self-image and confidence, and does not need time to reflect on her past problems and feelings.

   Option C: This may well be a correct activity for Susan at a later stage in the care programme. Currently she requires an activity which is more associated with the dissipation of energy.

   Option D   may again be suitable, but would be more appropriate at a later stage in the process of development.

3. There is an implication here that Susan's parents are worried about how they have failed in their responsibilities and also what other people may think of them.
   The response of the nurse, therefore, should be one which indicates to the parents the nurse's understanding of their situation, and willingness to discuss it with them.

   Option D is the correct response as it suggests a caring, accepting approach along with a willingness to discuss the matter further.

   Option A: This response accepts that Susan's parents have feelings about their daughter's situation but proceeds to close the door on further discussion. By making such a statement the nurse is probably pacifying herself more than she is helping or supporting the parents.

Option B: Similar to option A, the first part of this response is better in terms of displaying understanding; however, it still proceeds to suggest that there is nothing else to discuss.

Option C: It would be the responsibility of a skilled professional to try to explore these feelings a little more and offer support; if these strategies were unsuccessful then the situation could be referred to another helper.

4. The experiences which can damage an individual's trust and confidence in interpersonal relationships are inconsistency, unreliability, criticism and dishonesty. In order to re-establish a trusting relationship the nurse should display and use those qualities and skills which counter such experiences.

Option D is therefore the correct response.

Options A, B and C: All contain the skill of encouragement; whilst this may be worthwhile in other contexts, it is inappropriate in the development of trust and confidence.

5. One way of assisting Susan would be to help her to examine her behaviours and feelings. In this way it is hoped that she will develop a better understanding of herself and the rationale for her behaviour.

Option A is the correct response. Open-ended questions prevent the use of monosyllabic answers. This technique thus encourages the individual to talk, and in so doing provides opportunities to discuss and examine emotional reactions.

Options B and C: Both indicate something about the qualities of the nurse and are useful in relationship and interactive situations: however, they do not provide the best method for exploration.

Option D: suggests that time alone is the best method. Time is, of course, essential, but the quality of the interactions is of greater value than the time itself.

6. All of the options are examples of responding skills. As such, they are used in counselling situations and indicate to the client that the nurse is interested and listening. Additionally the use of these skills encourages the client to continue.

Option C is the correct response. Reflecting means feeding back to the client the words spoken and the observed feelings associated with them.

Option A: Paraphrasing is when the counsellor re-phrases or rewords the significant point of an interaction.

Option B: Clarification is the process of asking the client to explain her meaning of a particular word or phrase, or give specific examples of situations in order that the counsellor is not guessing at meanings.

Option D: Summarising may be carried out periodically or at the end of a session, and allows the counsellor to give a synopsis of the salient features so far and also to look forward to subsequent sessions.

7. The move from dependence to independence is a complex and frightening process. The role of the nurse is to guide Susan through this time of insecurity.

Option A is the correct response. Susan will require support whilst experimenting with new behaviours, and encouragement to persevere when situations become difficult. Education and counselling are required in order that Susan can develop self-awareness and explore alternative coping strategies. Within this process other skills will of course be employed.

Options B, C and D: All contain the skill of instructing. Although this can be seen as a method of education, it is of a directive type. A requirement for Susan is to develop an 'independent life-style': instruction would be more likely to foster dependence rather than independence.

8. Observation is a difficult yet essential responsibility of the nurse. When considering the possibility of self-harm, 'discreet' observation is often discussed. It is the belief of the authors that such a type of observation is almost impossible to carry out and often creates feelings of suspicion and resentment when the observation is denied by the nurse.

Option B is the correct response. It is a mature and client-involved statement which demonstrates the nurse's feelings for Susan and her acceptance of these feelings.

Option A may indeed be true; however, it is not an honest answer to Susan's straightforward question.

Option C: With this type of response the nurse is merely trying to avoid any confrontation; by giving an answer which is not honest the nurse is likely to disturb any relationship thus far developed.

Option D: Here the nurse is attempting to deflect the subject to an area which she wishes to talk about, rather than discuss the subject which is concerning Susan.

9. Susan has demonstrated on a number of occasions in her life that she is a vulnerable person. As she proceeds through therapy some difficult issues will be raised and she will need help to confront them.

Option D is the correct response.

Option A: This is of course correct but does not give any indication as to why support would be required during therapy.

Option B: This again is true; however, it relates to her past behaviours. The nurse should acknowledge such details and use them in the present to help Susan whilst she is undergoing therapy.

Option C: This would be an unfortunate consequence of inadequate support but is not the main reason why support should be provided.

Essay questions

1. Susan has recently been transferred to an acute psychiatric unit from a medical ward where she was admitted after taking 15–20 aspirin tablets.

   She has been experiencing relationship difficulties with her boyfriend and 3 months ago they separated. Since that time she has lost interest in herself and the care of her 8-year-old daughter.

   A Describe how the nurse should attempt to initiate and maintain a relationship with Susan.   25%

   B Explain the skills which might be used by the nurse to assist Susan to work through her feelings regarding her daughter.   25%

   C Describe the role of the nurse in assisting Susan to develop an independent life-style.   50%

2. Susan is a 34-year-old ex-nurse. Following the end of a long-term relationship she attempted to take her own life by ingesting 15–20 aspirin tablets. She was admitted to a medical ward where her physical condition was stabilised, she was then transferred to an acute psychiatric unit.

   A Describe skills which may be used by the nurse to reduce the possibility of further attempts at suicide   70%

   B Give, with explanations, an example of how the nurse should respond after one week of contact, if Susan states: 'I don't know why you are bothering, nobody wants me anymore anyway, I'm not worried whether I live or die.'   30%

3. Susan has recently been transferred from a medical ward. Three months ago her boyfriend with whom she had lived for 12 years, walked out on the relationship. Since that time she has gradually lost interest in everything around her. This culminated in an attempt to take her own life by ingesting 15–20 aspirin tablets. Following detoxification she was transferred to an acute psychiatric ward.

   A Describe the processes of reacting to loss, with particular reference to Susan's behaviour.   15%

   B Describe techniques which the nurse could use to assist this lady to adjust to her loss.   55%

   C How may the nursing staff help Susan's parents at this time?   30%

Specimen answer

1. A The nurse should be aware of the importance of the initial contact with Susan in terms of displaying genuineness, a feeling of warmth and a non-judgemental approach: she should be aware throughout of the non-verbal communications of both herself and the client.

   For the maintenance of the relationship, the behaviours and interventions of the nurse should demonstrate reliability, honesty, consistency, maturity and a willingness to invest time in Susan.

   B For Susan to work through her guilt feelings it will be necessary for the nurse to use the following skills:
   — sensitivity to Susan's feelings
   — responding skills which would encourage ventilation:
       open-ended questions, reflecting, paraphrasing, clarifying.
   — guidance skills to encourage Susan to identify:
       specific feelings and problems
       choice of strategies related to feelings or problems
       choice of particular strategy appropriate to her needs.
   — non-verbal communication as a means of encouraging ventilation or to offer support throughout this process.

   C   In developing an independent life-style Susan should be helped to work through the following processes:
   — self-development: an examination is required of her characteristics, philosophy and aims of life.
   — occupation of time: both leisure and work
   — management of time, finance and accommodation.
       To facilitate these processes the nurse needs to utilise a variety of skills:
   — guiding and educating, giving information, identifying problems and exploring strategies
   — counselling, using such skills as clarifying and challenging
   — group facilitating as a method of helping Susan's personal development
   — liaising with other health professionals or outside agencies
   — encouraging through difficult processes and offering feedback
   — supporting during testing out and gradual increase in Susan's personal responsibility.

Answer guides

2. A Relationship skills:
   — developing and maintaining trust
   — acceptance
   — consistency
   — reliability
   — honesty.

Counselling skills:
— encourage exploration of feelings
— work through problems, encourage realism.
Observational skills:
— patient involvement
— reduce harmful situations
— explanations to others.
Planning skills:
— client involvement
— setting goals.
Developing self-confidence, self-image:
— discussion
— choice of activities
— guidance about appearance
— encouragement.
Support:
— verbal and non-verbal
— short and long term.

B The following are examples of responses that could be made: 'What makes you feel that you are not worth bothering about?' or 'You seem to feel lost and uncertain at the moment, why do you think that you are not worth bothering about?'

This type of response will encourage Susan to go further in the expression of her feelings. She may then feel some benefit through catharsis or through the opportunity to explore her feelings and responses. The nurse would also demonstrate her acceptance of Susan's need to check out her feelings, and be offering support in a mature way.

Responses which attempt to confirm to Susan that she is still worth bothering with, e.g., 'Of course people still want you', are not acceptable in this situation. Such responses only serve the needs of the insecure nurse by limiting the discussion, and almost deny Susan the right to have or to explore these feelings.

3. A The following table outlines the links between the stages of the grieving process and Susan's behaviour.

Stages	Explanation of what these terms mean in the context of loss	Evident in Susan's *behaviour*
Denial		No—although this may have occurred.
Bargaining		Yes evidence to
Anger		Yes support these
Depression		Yes beliefs.
Acceptance		No

B The concentration of the nurse should be focussed on the processes
  employed in assisting Susan to adjust to this loss.
  Relationship formation:
  — honesty, consistency, reliability and genuineness.
  Counselling skills:
  — encourage ventilation, exploration and catharsis.
  Facilitation skills:
  — assisting Susan to identify problems, goals and strategies
  — assisting Susan to re-establish self-image and confidence:
      role play techniques could be included as part of this process
      stimulation and involvement in other activities.
  Encouragement:
  — to persevere during difficulties. The use of verbal and social reinforcers
    may be of value, providing that a therapeutic relationship has been
    established.
  Support:
  — employing verbal and non-verbal techniques.
  Attention should also be given to accommodation, financial and family
  difficulties.

C The first step is to establish the needs of Susan's parents at this time. This
  should then lead to an identification and use of the following skills:
  Relationship formation:
  — availability, approachability, concern and warmth.
  Interviewing:
  — establish the setting
  — explain the purpose
  — questioning technique
  — listening.
  Counselling:
  — encourage ventilation and discussion of feelings through responding
    techniques and non-judgemental acceptance.
  Supporting:
  — use of verbal and non-verbal techniques.
  Facilitating:
  — arranging facilitated discussion sessions
  — act as intermediary and negotiator between Susan and her parents.

7. Disruptive personal life-style associated with antisocial behaviour

Billy Johnson is 22 years of age, the youngest of five brothers. He drifts in and out of jobs and relationships and has a history of violent and impulsive behaviour especially when drunk. He tends to be self-centred and lacks control. At times he resorts to aggression in order to satisfy his needs and at other times he is manipulative.

His father left home when he was 3 years old and was succeeded in the household by a number of live-in boyfriends, some of whom treated Billy badly. Gradually his mother started drinking to excess and became dependent on tranquillisers. She died when Billy was 8 years of age and he was subsequently taken into care. From then until he was 16 he lived in a series of homes, some residential and some with foster parents. Few of these proved successful.

Billy's behaviour was described as disruptive and lacking in control. Since his admission, arguments and disruption have increased amongst the patients and staff. Billy appears to be central to these situations.

Multiple choice questions

1. Which one of the following offers the most accepted explanation of 'labelling'?
   A A system of categorising individuals into diagnostic groups for research and treatment.
   B A process in which an individual adopts for himself a certain status.
   C A system whereby deviant members of a society can recognise each other.
   D A process whereby society makes certain rules and classifies as deviant those who break them.

2. Which one of the following groups contains observations which would all suggest a diagnosis of psychopathic disorder?
   A Low tolerance to frustration, dulling of emotional response and demands for immediate gratification of needs.
   B Dulling of emotional response, demands for immediate gratification of needs and manipulative behaviour.
   C Demands for immediate gratification of needs, manipulative behaviour and low tolerance to frustration.
   D Manipulative behaviour, low tolerance to frustration and dulling of emotional response.

3. Which one of the following nursing actions would it be appropriate to take in response to Billy's attempts to manipulate nursing staff? The nurse should:
   A bring the behaviour to the attention of the ward community.
   B inform Billy of her feelings regarding the behaviour.
   C press Billy for explanations and justifications.
   D seek an apology from Billy.

4. Which one of the following groups contains principles which would all be appropriate to a limit-setting regime? That the limits set should be:
   A known to all, enforced consistently and related to the patient's background.
   B enforced consistently, related to patient's background and discussed with the patient.
   C related to the patient's background, discussed with the patient and known to all.
   D discussed with the patient, known to all and enforced consistently.

5. Which one of the following groups contains observations, made of Billy, which would all suggest that the risk of a physical attack was increasing?
   A Increase in motor restlessness, expanding demand for personal space, and adoption of fixed, rigid postures.
   B Expanding demand for personal space, adoption of fixed, rigid postures, and use of clipped, harsh speech.
   C Adoption of fixed, rigid postures, use of clipped harsh speech, and increase in motor restlessness.
   D Use of clipped, harsh speech, increase in motor restlessness, and expanding demand for personal space.

6. Which one of the following groups of nursing actions would all be appropriate in managing a violent attack by Billy?
   A Use a number of nurses to effect restraint, continue to talk to him during restraint and take him to the ground as quickly as possible.
   B Continue to talk to him during restraint, take him to the ground as quickly as possible and restrain him by firmly holding his hands and feet.
   C Take him to the ground as quickly as possible, restrain him by firmly holding his hands and feet and use a number of nurses to effect restraint.
   D Restrain him by firmly holding his hands and feet, use a number of nurses to effect restraint and continue to talk to him during restraint.

7. Which one of the following nursing interventions would be appropriate if Billy threatens violence?
   A Allow him to ventilate anger.
   B Provide diversion or distraction.
   C Ignore the behaviour.
   D Reward any socially acceptable behaviour.

8. Which one of the following groups contains interventions which would all form part of an anger management programme for Billy?
   A Increase his verbal fluency, help him develop an understanding of the relationship between trigger factors and the physical experience of anger, and offer a relationship dependent on his behaviour.
   B Help him develop an understanding of the relationship between trigger factors and the physical experience of anger, help him to learn alternative responses to anger, and increase his verbal fluency.
   C Help him to learn alternative responses to anger, increase his verbal fluency and offer a relationship dependent on his behaviour.
   D Offer a relationship dependent on his behaviour, help him to learn alternative responses to anger, and help him develop an understanding of the relationship between trigger factors and the physical experience of anger.

9. Which one of the following groups contains interventions which could all help Billy to develop a more mature behaviour pattern?
   A Offer a relationship which encourages reparenting, reward acceptable and punish non-acceptable behaviour, and give direct and immediate feedback on his behaviour.
   B Reward acceptable and punish non-acceptable behaviour, give direct and immediate feedback on his behaviour, and accept the person but put limits on the behaviour.
   C Give direct and immediate feedback on his behaviour, accept the person but put limits on the behaviour and offer a relationship which encourages reparenting.
   D Accept the person but put limits on the behaviour, offer a relationship which encourages reparenting, and reward acceptable and punish non-acceptable behaviour.

Answer keys to MCQs

1. Labelling is an important concept in the sociology of mental health and mental illness and can have profound effects on a client's behaviour and life-style.

   Option D is the correct response. It recognises that the labelling is socially determined and stems initially from society adopting and conforming to certain rules and customs. These rules or codes of conduct can be unwritten but may also be legitimised or made formal within the legal framework. Individuals who break these rules are classed as deviant and become stigmatised. In a way they are set aside from society generally, and their deviant influence is thus minimised.

   The process may also serve to reinforce the concept of conformity and reduce the temptation for others to behave in nonconformist ways.

   In some ways it is akin to scapegoating in that all the problems of society can be ascribed to the deviants, thereby reducing the pressure on responsible agencies to tackle the fundamental causes rather than the effects.

   The individual classed as deviant may well suffer from rejection and ostracism and be forced into closer contact with other deviants. This leads to a process of deviance amplification and adoption of the mores or rules of conduct of a deviant sub-culture.

   Option A is medically orientated using concepts of diagnosis and treatment. Labelling is a process occurring within society at large and can be seen in such labels as delinquent, drop-out or down-and-outs, and not just in psychiatric or medical labels.

   Option B recognises the deviance amplification and the transition into a deviant sub-culture with a different set of rewards and expectations. There is no recognition, however, that it is society and not the individual who does the labelling.

   Option C includes some elements of the deviant sub-culture. As individuals become classed as deviant so they may adopt standards of dress and behaviour which contribute to this self-image of being 'different' and may also help them to maintain a corporate identity. This process is seen in many other areas of society, and whilst certain collective names may be used, i.e., football supporters, Rastafarians, ramblers, these names do not constitute labelling as such.

2. The term psychopathic disorder is not one that is universally accepted. The use of the word diagnosis suggests illness, a concept which has raised much debate in this field. However, both the term and its medical orientation will feature in the work of the psychiatric nurse.

Option C is the correct response. Those people who have been diagnosed as having some form of psychopathic disorder are likely to show all of the stated features.

The demands for instant fulfilment of needs and an inability to recognise the needs of others are noticeable. This leads to the other two features. Where needs are not instantly met, frustration arises and the individual may commit acts of an antisocial nature. The frustration tolerance is low and he may appear to be impulsive because of this. Over-concern with his own needs and an unwillingness to recognise those of others leads to manipulative behaviours, especially in cases where the needs cannot be fulfilled by demands based on aggression.

Options A, B and D: Contain a dulling of emotional response. This is common in many psychiatric disorders but the significant feature in psychopathic disorder is one of emotional over-responsiveness innappropriate to the situation.

3. Attempts at interpersonal manipulation are commonly met in working with clients who have low self-esteem and poor opinions of others.

Option B is the correct response. Here the nurse gives Billy non-defensive interpersonal feedback about his behaviour. This allows Billy to see his actions and its interpersonal consequences.

If done consistently, he may learn to adopt more effective ways of stating his needs. The nurse acts as a model for Billy in her open expression of feelings, without resorting to aggression or hostility. The nurse's recognition of the manipulative behaviour and her expression of that non-defensively does not reinforce the behaviour and may lead to its reduction.

Option A would be a viable proposition in a setting such as a therapeutic community. In such a situation all people involved are engaged in learning about their behaviours and trying out other ways of relating to people. In a general psychiatric ward this type of intervention may merely bring resentments and hostilities or serve to reinforce the behaviour through attention.

Option C It is quite likely that Billy has insufficient awareness to give explanations and justifications for his behaviour. Asking why people behaved in certain ways is seldom effective and usually results in defensiveness and an interference with an effective working relationship. The search for reasons is more likely to be related to the feelings of the nurse rather than those of the patient.

Option D This is another intervention based on the nurse's hurt feelings rather than Billy's needs. Apologies can be seen as humiliating, and if forced rather than offered have little or no value and merely lead to resentment.

4. If a limit-setting programme is to be successful then a number of principles and conditions must be met.

Option D is the correct response. All of the stated principles would be appropriate to a limit-setting programme. The limits must be discussed with the patient so that he has prior knowledge of expectations. This may help to avoid testing out behaviours in order to ascertain limits. In an ideal programme the patient's agreement would be gained regarding the limits, and contracts mutually agreed. In practice this is not always possible.

The limits must be known to all of those who come into contact with the patient in order to lessen the impact of manipulative behaviours and enable a consistency of approach.

The limits must then be enforced consistently and at the same time non-punitively. A consistent approach should reduce the incidence and impact of manipulative behaviours. Such a structure also provides a measure of security and control for the patient which may be needed in the initial stages of therapy.

Options A, B and C: contain reference to the patient's background. Limits should be set around what is reasonable and workable rather than vary according to the background of the patient.

5. A number of observations can be made of people when they become increasingly aroused, accelerating the risk of violence.

Option D is the correct response. All of the stated features would occur in increasing arousal.

Speech patterns change and the voice takes on a harsh and aggressive tone. Words become clipped and shortened and may be delivered in staccato form.

There is an increase in motor restlessness, the patient appearing 'jumpy' and unable to keep still. There may be elements within this of displacement activity as the person attempts to channel their increased arousal into areas other than fight or flight.

The demand for personal space will increase and invasions into that appear very threatening to the patient. Verbalisations to keep away or stay back may be consistent with this. The increase in demand for space can also be appreciated by nurses responsive and sensitive to interpersonal behaviours, at a level which is almost intuitive.

Options A, B and C: All include the adoption of fixed rigid postures. This is more characteristic of extreme fear and withdrawal rather than the build up to a physical attack.

6. Violent attacks are always serious. The risk of injury can be reduced, however, by following certain guidelines.

Option A is the correct response. All of the actions would be appropriate in managing a violent attack.

Restraint should, wherever possible, be effected by a number of nurses to reduce the likelihood of injury to both staff and patients. A number of nurses acting in a coordinated fashion can manage a violent situation in a secure and protected way, using the minimum of force and avoiding a protracted struggle.

Whilst the patient is being restrained, verbal interaction should be maintained in order to reassure the patient and to check out with him his feelings and level of control. Physical restraint should be relinquished as quickly as possible, and only through talking can the optimum time for this be judged.

Taking the patient to the ground reduces the potential for injury by lowering the force which he is able to exert. Whilst standing, a patient is able to lash out with fists, head and feet, but is far less able to do so on the ground. Restraining in this way should only be contemplated in extreme cases and not, for example, when a patient is merely verbally aggressive.

Options B, C and D: All contain restraint by firmly holding feet and hands. If physical restraint has to be effected then the patient should be held as near to major joints as possible and not by the extremities. Holding near joints reduces the leverage which can be exerted and therefore diminishes the risk of injury.

7. There are a number of possible interventions that can be made to reduce the likelihood of physical attack when a patient is threatening violence.

Option A is the correct response. The nurse should try at all times to allow the ventilation of anger rather than suppress it and then risk the expression of the anger through physical assault. The patient's statements, protestations and threats should be taken non-defensively, thus avoiding escalation. The nurse should enable the patient to 'back down' without loss of face. Whilst ventilating, the patient may be displacing the anger and working through the issue. Maintaining a dialogue allows the nurse to 'talk down' the patient from heightened states of arousal.

Option B is a possible intervention at an earlier stage. Providing a constructive outlet for energy may reduce its expression in aggression.

Option C Ignoring maladaptive behaviour may result in its eventual decrease. Threats of violence, however, are too serious to ignore.

Option D This style of management should be applied generally but is not an appropriate intervention for this specific incident.

8. A number of techniques can be made available for people to manage their anger more effectively. In many ways the process is similar to cognitive behaviour therapy for the management of anxiety.

Option B is the correct response. All of the interventions could form part of a programme dealing with anger management. The development of an understanding between external trigger factors and the internal experience of anger can help people to respond more appropriately to those situations. Many people with difficulties in this area can feel that they have no control over their reactions and that their behavioural response is almost automatic. Alternative ways of dealing with anger such as shouting or withdrawing and going for a walk may be learned and used in situations which have formerly elicited violence. Increasing verbal fluency may help people to state their needs and feelings more appropriately rather than resorting to violence as an outward expression of them.

Options A, C and D: All contain the offering of a relationship dependent on behaviour. The principle here should be to offer an unconditional approval of respect for the person but to set limits on the behaviour.

9. The adoption of immature patterns of behaviour is a fairly consistent feature of people with this sort of difficulty. A number of interventions may help people to work through their problems in this area.

Option C is the correct response. All of the interventions may prove useful. Feedback upon behaviour should be given in a direct, assertive and controlled fashion and should be given as soon after the incident as possible. The feedback should be aimed at an area which can be controlled and related to behaviour rather than personality characteristics. The relationship should be based upon acceptance or unconditional positive regard. At the same time limits upon acceptable and non-acceptable behaviours should be stated. A stable, firm, consistent but accepting relationship may allow Billy to work out some of his maturational difficulties with a parent figure which may have been lacking in the past.

Options A, B and D: All contain the reward of acceptable and punishment of non-acceptable behaviours. Punishment is seldom effective as a tool for changing behaviours. Indeed people such as Billy will be likely to have experienced punishment and rejection for a lot of their lives. Different strategies are required which allow people to work through their difficulties rather than being punished for them.

Essay questions

1. Billy, aged 22 years, is a recently admitted patient. He tends to be self-centred and lacking in personal control. He has a history of violent and impulsive behaviour.

   A Describe the principles which should underpin a limit-setting regime.   20%

   B Discuss a programme of anger management which could help Billy to exercise more control over his violent behaviour.   50%

   C Discuss possible attitudes of nursing staff towards Billy and his behaviour.   30%

2. Billy Johnson, aged 22 years, is the youngest of five brothers. His father left home when he was 3 years old and was succeeded in the household by a number of live-in boyfriends, some of whom treated Billy badly. His mother had a drink and drugs problem and died when he was 8. Subsequently Billy was in care and experienced a number of residential and foster homes.

   He has drifted in and out of jobs and relationships and has a history of violence especially when drunk. He was admitted to an acute psychiatric unit where his behaviour was described as aggressive and manipulative.

   A Discuss measures which could have been taken in the past which might have helped Billy to develop a more positive life-style.   40%

   B Describe nursing approaches which would help Billy with the difficulties he is experiencing.   60%

3. Billy Johnson, aged 22 years, is a recently admitted patient with a history of antisocial behaviour. At times he resorts to aggression in order to satisfy his needs and at other times he is manipulative.

   Since his admission, arguments and disruption have increased amongst the ward community, with Billy apparently playing a central part in these situations.

   A Outline the possible causes for the increased incidence of these situations.   20%

   B Describe nursing interventions which will help the ward community to resolve these problems.   40%

   C Discuss the nursing strategy which should operate during Billy's early care.   40%

Specimen answer

1. A A major principle in a limit-setting regime is that of making the expectations clear and explicit. Ideally, the standards of acceptable behaviour should be mutually agreed between staff and patient. These limits should be known and enforced consistently by all health care personnel.

The limits applied to behaviours should be reasonable and restricted to those which clearly impinge upon the rights and interests of others. Empty threats or promises reinforce the patient's views that others cannot be depended upon. The means of enforcing the limits must be available and feasible.

In enforcing the limits the nurse should remain calm, assertive, in control and avoid arguments which belittle the client. Engaging in accusations and demanding justifications are futile, and all elements of a power struggle should be avoided.

B There are two major components to anger. The first is an affective component concerned with emotional arousal and the second is a cognitive component concerned with thoughts, expectations and attentional processes. These are intimately connected so that what people think in given situations can escalate the way that they feel. The increased arousal may also affect cognitive and judgemental processes leading to a violent attack.

A programme of anger management must address both issues. It may start with an exploration and understanding of particular situations causing arousal. These triggers should be linked to feelings and thoughts. The object is to break down the response into component parts which can then be dealt with and the anger understood in terms of a number of phases rather than an all-or-nothing response.

The cognitive functions can be changed by enabling clients to understand the self-statements that they make when faced with a stressor and to change those to statements of coping and control.

The arousal can be reduced by applying relaxation and other diversional or channelling skills. These are similar in many ways to those used in stress reduction for anxiety and must be worked out on an individual basis.

The stressor can be utilised as the cue for engaging in problem-solving and the techniques of that can be learnt. Social skills training and particularly the skills of behaving assertively can be learnt and used when the situation demands.

C The attitudes of nursing staff may be both positive and negative.

On the positive side nurses may have realistic expectations and a positive desire to help. They will be mature in outlook and aware of themselves and their own needs. They must be capable of remaining assertive in the face of aggressive and manipulative behaviours and should be able to offer acceptance and regard for the client without condoning or attacking his aberrant behaviours.

There are many negative attitudes which may be elicited from nursing staff by these behaviours. Mainly, these are motivated by fears and resentments and expressed in hostility, rejection, scapegoating and other such behaviours.

Answer guides

2. A Measures which could have been taken:
   — early intervention by health care agencies to provide support, case-work for mother and a stable home environment for Billy.
   — recognition and provision of an environment which offered love, caring, stability and physical care.
   — interventions by agencies at school, i.e., school nurse, child guidance, educational psychologist.
   — placement of Billy in a consistent home.
   — help for Billy during adolescence from child care agencies.
   — support, guidance and friendship as Billy goes out to work.
   — recognition by authorities of Billy's emotional needs and help with problems of early adult life.

   B Nursing approaches:
   — provision of a stable relationship which is accepting but firm, consistent and caring, and offers an opportunity to learn from a significant adult those things which he should have learnt through contact with a parent.
   — modelling of open expression of needs, feelings and assertive behaviours.
   — clear and direct feedback to Billy about his behaviour.
   — limit-setting regimes.
   — programmes of anger management.
   — training in assertiveness and other social skills.

3. A The possible causes of the increase could include:
   — Billy behaving in manipulative and aggressive ways in order to satisfy his own needs or as a response to authority or lack of freedom.
   — other patients being manipulated or cowed by Billy's behaviour leading to the expression of their feelings in covert ways rather than openly.
   — staff reactions to Billy. Projection of fears and anger onto other staff, patients or situations rather than dealing with the underlying issues of authority and power.

   B Interventions with Billy:
   — help him to understand and work through his problems.
   — offer help through counselling and skills training.
   — explore Billy's reaction to hospitalisation and enforced routines and procedures.
   — offer alternative ways of dealing with the issues.
   Interventions for staff:
   — staff meetings to reach a consensus on ways of responding to Billy.

— offer support and supervision, training and feedback especially for junior staff.
— allow the free expression of feelings both positive and negative.
Interventions for other patients:
— meetings to air grievances, fears and misunderstandings.
— offer individual help where necessary.

C Explore his reactions to hospital and the reason for his admission.
Help him to reach some understanding regarding problem ownership.
Involve him in discussion about limits, behaviour and contracts.
Discuss the nature of the relationship and how limits will be enforced. Check for understanding.
Reach consensus and agreements with staff regarding limit-setting programme.
Ensure consistency of approach.
Allow time and opportunity for him to air fears and grievances.
Engage him in assessment of needs and problem areas.

8. Disruptive personal life-style associated with alcohol

Bob Younger is a 37-year-old married man who has been advised to seek help because of problems he is experiencing associated with alcohol abuse.

There is no psychiatric or significant medical history concerning either of his parents who are both retired school teachers. He has one older brother who is also alive and well.

On leaving school he gained employment as a bricklayer's labourer but left this after 3 years to take up his present job as a sales representative. A car was supplied with this job which he saw as a significant attraction.

Whilst working as a labourer he met his future wife. They had an on/off relationship for approximately 1 year, following which they became more serious. This lasted for 12 months after which they were married. They have now been married for 17 years and have four children whose ages range from 5 to 16 years.

His first serious drinking sessions started just before he left school; he then progressed into regular social drinking whilst working on building sites. His wife states that he was drinking quite heavily on occasions, even at that time.

His drinking caused friction in their relationship. In turn, the friction made the drinking problem worse. Bob argues that he preferred to stay out late at night drinking with his friends rather than returning home to face more arguments.

He agrees that his consumption has increased significantly over the past 2 years to approximately 30 units of alcohol per day. As a result of a breath test he lost his driving licence and consequently his job is now in jeopardy.

His wife says that she did not know what to do for the best; in desperation she rang the General practitioner and through their joint efforts at persuasion, Bob reluctantly agreed to an out-patient appointment and subsequent admission to hospital, although he continued to maintain that he was in control of his drinking.

In hospital he was initially helped through a 1 week period of detoxification and is at the moment undergoing a care programme which involves the use of intensive group therapy.

Multiple choice questions

1. Which one of the following groups of needs would be experienced by Bob whilst he withdraws from alcohol?
   A Security, safety, nutrition, rehydration and rest.
   B Safety, nutrition, rehydration, rest and coping skills.
   C Nutrition, rehydration, rest, coping skills and security.
   D Rehydration, rest, coping skills, security and safety.

2. Which one of the following groups of nursing skills would be appropriate when caring for Bob during withdrawal from alcohol?
   A Communication, education and reassurance.
   B Education, reassurance and encouragement.
   C Reassurance, encouragement and communication.
   D Encouragement, communication and education.

3. Which one of the following groups of nursing objectives would help Bob to resolve his problems, following withdrawal from alcohol?
   A Provide support, increase his self-esteem, develop his coping skills and encourage realistic goal setting.
   B Increase his self-esteem, develop his coping skills, encourage realistic goal setting and provide stimulation.
   C Develop his coping skills, encourage realistic goal setting, provide stimulation and provide support.
   D Encourage realistic goal setting, provide stimulation, provide support and increase his self-esteem.

4. Which one of the following would be the first aim in Bob's long-term care following withdrawal from alcohol?
   A Ensure that he feels supported by both staff and family.
   B Set realistic goals for his care.
   C Increase his self-awareness and self-confidence.
   D Bob's acceptance that he has a problem with his drinking.

5. Which one of the following statements by Bob most clearly indicates that his motivation to resolve his problems is realistic?
   A 'I must stop in order to keep my job.'
   B 'I just want to be able to drink normally again.'
   C 'I want to stop for my own peace of mind.'
   D 'I must stop for the sake of my wife and children.'

6. Which one of the following groups contains the most appropriate range of skills the nurse could use when helping Bob adjust to his problems?
   A Encouragement, support, relationship formation, shaping and education.
   B Support, relationship formation, shaping, education and modelling.
   C Education, modelling, encouragement, support and relationship formation.
   D Modelling, encouragement, support, relationship formation and shaping.

7. Which one of the following contains 'processes' by which group therapy is believed to be effective?
   A Support, not feeling unique, increase self-awareness and cohesion.
   B Not feeling unique, increase self-awareness, cohesion and promoting catharsis.
   C Increase self-awareness, cohesion, promoting catharsis and support.
   D Cohesion, promoting catharsis, support and not feeling unique.

8. Which one of the following gives the most appropriate response of the group leader if Bob becomes tearful and angry whilst relating personal details to the group in his third session?
   A Suggest that he might feel better if he changes the subject for the moment.
   B Point out that the group would like him to continue when his tears are finished.
   C Initially say nothing; if no other member comments then explain that it is alright to display emotion.
   D Ask other group members to give their interpretation of what is happening.

9. Which one of the following groups contains services which would offer the best long-term support for Bob and his family?
   A Alcoholics Anonymous, Al-anon, Cyrenians and social work.
   B Al-anon, Cyrenians, social work and significant phone numbers.
   C Cyrenians, social work, significant phone numbers and Alcoholics Anonymous.
   D Social work, significant phone numbers, Alcoholics Anonymous and Al-anon.

Answer keys to MCQs

1. Whilst Bob is withdrawing from alcohol the main principle of care must be to ensure his safety and general comfort.

   Option A is therefore the correct response.

   Options B, C and D: All include the development of coping skills and whilst this is likely to be a long-term goal it would be inappropriate at this stage of Bob's care.

2. During the withdrawal phase it is important that the reactions and skills of the nurse are appropriate to Bob's needs. At this time these will relate to his physical and emotional state.

   Option C is the correct response. Bob may well be experiencing anxiety, he will also require a great deal of encouragement even with such basic functions as eating. Because withdrawal produces degrees of disorientation and perceptual distortion, communication skills are a necessary attribute.

   Options A, B and D: All include the use of educational skills. Although these will undoubtedly be used during the later stages of care they are unlikely to be of any real value during the withdrawal phase.

3. As the client moves from the process of detoxification his needs will become more related to ways in which he can maintain his abstinence. For this to occur Bob will need to establish goals which are realistic, re-develop his self-esteem and confidence and identify alternative coping strategies. Throughout this difficult process he will require a great deal of support.

   Option A is the correct response.

   Options B, C and D: All suggest the need for stimulation. This is indeed considered to be a human need. However, related to the feelings an alcoholic has about himself, and the work in therapy which Bob is about to undertake, it is not a major factor at this time.

4. One device used by the human mind in order to protect its self-image is the process of denial. It is a process which can be seen in many situations ranging from bereavement to being confronted by the suggestion that one might be an alcoholic. Often if the reasons for the admission of alcoholics are studied, it can be seen, as with Bob, that the admission process is a reluctant one, rather than one that is agreed to with a view to resolving problems.

   Option D is the correct response. Bob's cooperation in therapy is essential, without this all other measures will almost certainly fail.

Options A, B and C: All of these factors are important. However in a priority listing, acceptance of the problem is the first aim; hence the introduction one often hears from alcoholics, 'Hello, I'm Bob. I'm an alcoholic.'

5. In attempting to help the client resolve his problems, 'success' is more likely if it can be deduced that his level of motivation is high. This is a difficult area to assess but one which is not indicated by the expression of fanciful ideas or over-commitment to other people as the reason for stopping drinking.

Option C is the correct response as it indicates that Bob wishes to stop drinking and wants to do so for himself. If other people derive benefit from this, it is initially a secondary consideration.

Option A: If this is the motivating force then the client is not likely to resolve his problems. Indeed, if he discovered that he could not retain his employment then, in effect, his reason for not drinking will have been removed.

Option B: A common desire in any person who experiences problems with his drinking: however, there is evidence to suggest that if the drinker is not young or has experienced physical withdrawal symptoms, he is more likely to relapse under a controlled drinking regime.

Option D: As indicated in other options, in the first instance Bob must want to stop drinking for himself.

6. When Bob enters the phase of therapy where he is working towards resolving his difficulties, he will be learning about alcohol and about himself. He will explore what makes him what he is, his reactions, strengths and weaknesses. The prospect of this process is a daunting one, which most people would approach with some trepidation.

Option C is the correct response as all the skills would be of value in helping the client through this process.

Options A, B and D: All contain the process of shaping. This is a valid technique which may be employed by the nurse therapist but not in response to Bob's problems.

7. Group processes are the ways in which a psychotherapy group is believed to exert its effect. They are the means by which a group achieves its aims. They are not the aims themselves, nor are they tasks which a group may be expected to carry out as part of its functioning.

Option D is the correct response.

Options A, B and C: All include the aim to increase self-awareness. This is
something which Bob would hope to achieve through the group. It is,
therefore, more realistically an aim rather than a group process.

8. In the early stages of the group the leader should encourage the members to
set the climate of work, one which is productive, yet safe to express personal
feelings.

Option C allows individual group members to respond to Bob's feelings but
gives the leader the opportunity to promote the understanding that
such a display of feelings is acceptable.

Option A would ensure the safety of the client but would also encourage in
him the idea that if a situation becomes difficult it can be avoided.

Option B is acceptable but at a later stage in the development of the group, or
in Bob's therapy, when the group has learned to face situations of
confrontation.

Option D is again an acceptable response, but is more appropriate at a later
stage in the life of the group.

9. In order to enhance the prospects for long-term recovery it is essential that
adequate support services be offered, not merely to the client but also to his
family. Following the withdrawal of active day-to-day support and almost
constant supervision this family may experience many difficulties.

Option D is the correct response. All of these agencies would be appropriate,
considering the difficulties which may be encountered by Bob and his
family.

Options A, B and C: All include the offer of help from the Cyrenians. This is an
organisation which provides help predominantly to homeless
alcoholics, and is therefore not applicable to Bob.

Essay questions

1. Bob Younger has recently been admitted to hospital for help with an alcohol problem. Initially he was helped through the process of detoxification.
   A How should the nursing team assess the needs/problems of the client following the process of detoxification? 30%
   B How can the nursing staff help Bob to work towards a life without alcohol, and what skills should the nurse use to facilitate this change? 70%

2. Bob is 37 years old and has recently been admitted to hospital because he is experiencing problems with alcohol. He is married and has four children whose ages range from 5 to 16 years.
   A Discuss the possible effects of Bob's drinking on the family. 15%
   B What advice and information should be given and discussed with the family? 55%
   C What should be the nurse's verbal response and why when Bob's wife says, 'I am not sure what to do for the best, nurse. I am frightened of what will happen when he comes home'? 30%

3. Bob has been admitted to hospital because he is experiencing problems with alcohol. Following a 2 week period of detoxification and assessment it has been recommended that he joins a psychotherapy group.
   A What should be the role of the nurse in leading group therapy sessions with individuals who are experiencing problems with alcohol? 30%
   B Explain the stages which the group would pass through in its development and how these would be recognised. 30%
   C In what ways would the group processes help this client in his efforts to come to terms with and resolve his problems? 40%

Specimen answer

1. A   Assessment should be carried out using the processes of observation, data collection and interviewing.

   By observing such things as the physical well-being and social interaction of the client, it may be possible to identify areas of difficulty.

   The interview process is an important tool and will enable the nurse to explore with Bob and his family their beliefs about the problems, expectations and difficulties related to his condition.

   Data collection is the process whereby information obtained by other personnel is brought together and examined for significant factors.

   It is important to involve the client and his family in the identification of problems to ensure that all those involved actually agree on the nature of their problems.

   B   The first stage in helping Bob work towards a life without alcohol is to identify his perceptions of the problems. This can be achieved in the ways outlined above.

   When this has been achieved it is essential to move into the area of problem acceptance, in other words to help Bob come to terms with the fact that he has a problem with alcohol. This is likely to be a difficult area as he has only reluctantly agreed to the offer of help. Whether in groups or individually, the nurse must discuss the whole question of alcohol, problem drinking and definitions of alcoholism, in order to help him accept his own problems within these areas.

   A great deal of support will be necessary during this process and through the subsequent weeks of work. The nurse may best help the client at this time by giving of the self, active listening, and the expression of verbal support. Through these means Bob may come to feel accepted and not left to face his problems alone.

   Throughout this process a relationship will be developing. The nurse must endeavour to be honest, open and consistent to establish a mature relationship. The nurse must also be realistic, and be prepared to confront Bob regarding aspects of his behaviour or information which are inconsistent.

   One of the difficulties which Bob is likely to face is the setting of realistic goals. Here the nurse can help through facilitating the examination of his life and expectations. This is an area which will be helped by their developing relationship and the nurse's ability to offer support.

   The nurse will require counselling skills in order to help the client to ventilate his feelings and emotions. This may be achieved on an individual basis or through group work. Counselling skills are also likely to be of benefit during discussions with Bob's wife. When dealing with her, and perhaps the older child, some educational skills may be needed. These can be used in much the same way as with Bob, to examine their perceptions of alcohol and problem drinking. Group work skills are also necessary as Bob is undergoing intensive group therapy. These skills should include the ability to establish a group, its climate and aims. When the group is operating the nurse must display the ability to monitor objectively the processes of the group and direct the members to use the processes in order to examine themselves and their difficulties.

It is also important to use educational, supportive and encouraging skills to assist the client to examine his own life skills and those activities or facilities which may be of value to him.

As a final and essential area, long-term support must be discussed with Bob and his family; using supportive and educational skills the nurse should encourage Bob to make the right choices for his long-term future.

Answer guides

2. A Feelings of isolation: because of the social image of individuals with alcohol problems and their unreliability, the family, either enforced or voluntarily, may experience feelings of isolation.

Lack of understanding and knowledge of what makes an 'alcoholic'. For a variety of reasons the family may experience feelings of guilt and frustration.

Disturbed family relationships:

    effects upon wife:
    — mistrust
    — anger
    — frustration
    — loneliness.

    effects upon children:
    — mistrust
    — school problems
    — fear.

    effects upon Bob:
    — guilt
    — anger
    — jealousy
    — poor self-image.

B Over a period of time the following areas could be explored:
    — what is alcohol?
    — who is an alcoholic?
    — the care programme
    — the family's part in the recovery programme
    — warning signs of relapse
    — available support services for Bob and the family
    — advice on how the support services can be contacted
    — possible changes in the client's behaviour: has his wife known him when he has not been drinking heavily and what will be the effects of his abstinence?

— reactions of the children

— honesty with others.

C The type of response should be along the lines of: 'I understand that you feel apprehensive about this, perhaps we can look together at some of the concerns you have'.

In giving such a response the nurse is in effect saying to Bob's wife:

— It is alright to express your concern.

— I am willing to listen.

— Your reactions and feelings are understandable.

— Can you clarify specific areas of concern?

— You are not alone in trying to deal with these problems.

3. A The role would encompass the following elements:

Establishing the group:

— setting, frequency, time, open or closed, duration

— helping the group to determine its aims, norms and climate.

Maintaining the group:

— encourage group processes to occur

— reflect observations and information to the group in general

— some interpretation of processes and content may be appropriate.

Prepare for termination:

— allow as much time as possible

— repeat closing date of group (if appropriate) to clarify knowledge of members

— promote ventilation of feelings.

B A group will pass through a number of stages in its life: these are referred to in a variety of ways; however the behaviours remain the same. As group workers, it is more important to recognise the associated behaviours than specific terms of description.

Getting together:

— general introductions

— non-threatening conversations

— superficial discussion

— majority at pains not to disagree

— reliance upon the structure of a meeting, i.e., leaders leading.

Generalised feelings of insecurity:

— what are we doing here?

— anger directed at the leader

— behaviours aimed at testing the leadership

— conflict between individual members

Let's decide what we are doing:

— establishing rules and norms

— beginnings of positive confrontation

— individuals beginning to feel 'OK'.

Let's work together:
— expression of feelings
— differences of opinions
— working at own and other's problems
— offering support.
Time to leave:
— renewed feelings of insecurity
— individuals reflect on experiences shared by the group
— suggested reunions
— expressions of emotion about this event.

C   As group workers we must train ourselves to concentrate on what is happening within the group as opposed to merely listening to what is being said. In this way we can reflect or interpret our observations to the group. These processes are the ways in which the group is likely to be effective rather than through the content of discussions alone.

A feeling which is common to all individuals is that their problems are worse than those of anyone else. In a group situation Bob will find that he is meeting others experiencing similar difficulties.

It is hoped that a feeling of unity will develop in the group, leading to a bonding of individuals into the whole

Society's concept of alcohol and the disruptive nature of problem drinking cause many alcoholics to feel isolated and alone.

Optimism may gradually develop as the group reaches the stage of actually working on the problems of individual members.

The group may act as a pressure valve by allowing clients an opportunity to express their feelings.

Active support will be in evidence from the group as a whole: this is an essential process as Bob will have to face some difficult issues such as decision-making and examining himself and his life.

By practising the re-establishment of social relationships within the group, his self-image and self-esteem are likely to be enhanced.

In the group Bob will be able to examine his psychological make-up and his social and family relationships. As a consequence of this examination he may experiment with his communications and interactions and the group will provide a safe sounding board.

By a process of modelling, either conscious or unconscious, brought about by listening to other members discuss their problems and coping strategies, Bob may be helped to develop and attempt alternative coping behaviours of his own.

9. Loss of contact with reality associated with depression

David is 48 years old, married, and has three children, one of whom still lives at home.

According to his wife, David has led an uneventful life; leaving school with several qualifications he gained employment in the offices of a manufacturing company. It was here that he met his wife and they were married 26 years ago. David has no previous psychiatric history but his mother was treated for 'nerves' on two occasions when he was in his late teens. Over the past 6 months he has felt increasingly unwell, expressing great concern about his physical well-being; he now suspects that he may have a serious physical illness. He has difficulty in sustaining conversations, looks extremely sad and is expressing ideas about being a burden upon his family.

His wife points out that he has undoubtedly slowed down over the past 6 months. He appears to lack interest in virtually everything, has been forced to take sick leave from work and is a source of great concern for her.

Because his wife works and David would be alone for long periods during the day, it was felt advisable that he be admitted for psychiatric care. This was arranged voluntarily at the local psychiatric unit.

Multiple choice questions

1. Which one of the following groups of symptoms indicates that David was experiencing a severe type of depressive reaction?
   A Constipation, difficulty in falling asleep, slowness of actions and self-neglect.
   B Difficulty in falling asleep, slowness of actions, self-neglect and poverty of thought.
   C Slowness of actions, self-neglect, poverty of thought and constipation.
   D Self-neglect, poverty of thought, constipation and difficulty in falling asleep.

2. Which one of the following styles of communication should the nurse use if David displays a slowness of thinking in the early stages of his care?
   A Speak normally but explain that you understand his difficulty.
   B Communicate normally but do not move on to another topic until the previous question has been answered.
   C Include light-hearted topics and gestures which would serve as a role model.
   D Use short, non-patronising questions or statements and allow time for him to respond.

3. Which one of the following would be the most appropriate response for the nurse to make when David says, 'I don't know why you bother with me, nurse, I shouldn't be taking up your time'?
   A 'Don't talk like that David, you know I am here to help.'
   B 'It is no problem, I have plenty of time.'
   C 'But I want to bother, I really want to help you resolve your problems.'
   D 'You feel very low at the moment but I would like us to work together on how you are feeling.'

4. Which one of the following would be the best way for the nursing team to try and increase David's confidence and improve his self-perception?
   A Involve him in new, easily completed tasks.
   B Encourage him to try some old hobbies.
   C Involve him in group therapy.
   D Encourage him to carry out his family responsibilities.

5. Which one of the following would be the most appropriate action for the nurse to take, when, during a course of electro-convulsive therapy, David asks to speak with her about the treatment?
   A Be prepared to discuss honestly and openly those aspects of treatment which interest him.
   B Suggest that he is at liberty to know, but that the doctor is the best person to ask.
   C Explain that it is not really known how the treatment works, but that it is known to be effective.
   D Explain that he has a right to know, but perhaps it would be better to wait until he had improved a little.

6. Which one of the following would be the most appropriate action for the nurse to take if, shortly before he is due to receive electro-convulsive therapy, David informs the nurse that he was thirsty and has had a small drink of water?
   A Clarify with David the amount taken and allow treatment to proceed.
   B Validate the statement and inform the nurse in charge of treatment.
   C Clarify with David the amount consumed and arrange cancellation of the treatment.
   D Validate David's statement and explain to him that treatment will have to be postponed.

7. Which one of the following would be the most appropriate response for the nurse to make when David, whilst showing signs of improvement, says, 'My wife has not visited to-day, perhaps she is fed up with me'?

A 'Are you sure she said she would come to-day, maybe she is coming this evening.'

B 'I am sure she is not fed up with you; what would you like to do this afternoon if she does not come?'

C 'You seem to be blaming yourself for her not coming; perhaps we could identify other reasons.'

D 'You are obviously upset by her not coming, but I am sure that there will be a logical explanation.'

8. Which one of the following groups contains the most appropriate actions for the nurse to take if David is considered to be at risk of attempting suicide?

A Foster self-understanding, minimise available methods, ensure accurate observations and honestly explain actions.

B Minimise available methods, ensure accurate observations, honestly explain actions and divert thoughts to more positive areas.

C Ensure accurate observations, honestly explain actions, divert thoughts to more positive areas and foster self-understanding.

D Honestly explain actions, divert thoughts to more positive areas, foster self-understanding and minimise available methods.

9. Which one of the following groups provides the most likely indicators that David was experiencing unwanted effects from his tricyclic chemotherapy?

A Dry mouth, disturbed vision, headache and dizziness.

B Disturbed vision, headache, dizziness and urinary difficulties.

C Headache, dizziness, urinary difficulties and dry mouth.

D Dizziness, urinary difficulties, dry mouth and disturbed vision.

Answer keys to MCQs

1. Over the years various terms have been used to differentiate between the types of depressive reactions. Regardless of the specific names used some individuals seem to experience a reaction which retards both mental and physical functioning.

   Option C is the correct response.

   Options A, B and D: All include sleep difficulty. Whilst this is a common feature of all depressive reactions, clients experiencing a severe type of depression most often complain of difficulties during the night or early morning.

2. Slowing of the ability to assimilate information and formulate replies is a recognised feature of some depressive reactions. The nurse in communicating with such clients must acknowledge these problems and adjust her approach accordingly.

   Option D is the correct response.

   Option A   would indicate that the nurse understood what David was experiencing, but would not make communication any easier.

   Option B: Whilst it is essential to allow David time to answer, if the nurse were to adopt this approach it would be likely to increase his tension and feelings of inadequacy.

   Option C   should not be used as it will only serve to point out to David his low mood and thereby make him feel worse.

3. Statements such as this indicate the lowered self-esteem of the client, at the same time he is looking for support; to be effusive in these circumstances could be detrimental.

   Option D is the correct response. It is an attempt by the nurse to indicate her understanding of how he is feeling, whilst at the same time offering the support and willingness to invest herself in his care.

   Option A   is too offhand and suggests that David should not say such things as he should know that the nurse is there to help.

   Option B   concentrates only on the second half of David's statement and ignores the aspect relating to self-image.

   Option C   appears to be acceptable. However, it has been suggested that when relating to a client who has a lowered self-image, this approach may increase the guilt feelings in the client at taking up the time of the nurse.

4. When a person experiences a depressive reaction his negative thoughts about confidence, abilities and self-image are continually reinforced. Due to poor concentration and an expectation of failure, the person concerned finds himself living a self-fulfilling prophecy.

Option A is the correct response. The tasks chosen are within the client's capability but are new to his experience, thereby not offering any past reference points for negative comparison. By these means the nurse can use every opportunity to praise and encourage his achievements, irrespective of how small. These techniques can help to re-establish the confidence and self-image of the client.

Option B   may be an acceptable intervention to employ. However, there is a danger that David knows what he used to be able to achieve: his achievements in therapy will inevitably be compared to his past abilities.

Option C: Involvement in group therapy may be acceptable if the type of therapy is carefully selected. It is likely, however, that some of his confidence will need to be restored through one-to-one relationships before such a step is considered.

Option D: Re-establishment of his role within the family is an important long-term goal. It will be necessary to build up to this level gradually. The development of confidence will be achieved more effectively if he does not have such responsibilities thrust upon him at too early a stage in his care.

5. An individual undergoing any form of therapy will have concerns and questions. This is particularly true when the therapy has a kind of mystique, and involves a combination of anaesthesia and electrical stimulation. The fact that David has asked the nurse such a question does not necessarily imply anxiety; it could merely be a wish to know about aspects of care. It is important that the nurse responds to David in a mature and open manner, recognising his right to know.

Option A is the correct response.

Option B   accepts the right of the client to know but implies an inclination to avoid the responsibility for giving or reminding him of the information he seeks.

Option C   is an incorrect response. It involves an assumption on the part of the nurse of what the client wishes to discuss. His concern could be about anything related to this treatment such as, 'Can my wife visit after the treatment?'

Option D   is similar to option B. There is an acceptance of David's right to know
but an inclination to evade the issue until a later date. He has asked
because whatever it is, concerns him now: an answer given in 2
weeks would be of little value.

6. Such a statement by David may indicate several possibilities, that he is
concerned about the treatment, that he wishes treatment to be deferred, or that
he has misunderstood the information given to him regarding fasting. Each one
of these situations can be dealt with in their turn, but in the first instance the
nurse should ensure the safety of the client.

Option B   is the correct response. The initial action of the nurse should be to
validate the statement made. When this has been done the
information should be referred, through the nurse in charge of the
department, to the anaesthetist. With this information, a balanced
decision can be made regarding the wisdom of continuing with the
treatment.

Options A, C and D: are all possibilities. The nurse must clarify the situation
regarding whether or not David has consumed any liquid, and if so
how much. The details should then be referred to those in charge of
the treatment area for a decision to be made. Under these
circumstances the nurse should not make such a decision herself.

7. As David starts to improve, the nurse should enourage him to examine the
statements he makes which reflect or reinforce his negative self-image. This is
essentially the technique of cognitive therapy.

Option C   is the correct response. This is a stage of the process where the
client is asked to recognise that he is attributing all actions in a
negative way to himself. He is encouraged to look at alternative
explanations. This process is designed to break into the cycle of
negative thoughts, non-achievement, negative thoughts.

Option A: In making this response the nurse is ignoring the self-deprecating
content of David's statement.

Option B   is a response which is designed to improve the mood of the client in
the short-term. The nurse offers her interpretation and attempts to
divert his thoughts onto another topic. As in Option A, there is a
denial of David's feelings about himself.

Option D   shows a recognition of David's feelings but does not encourage him
to look at other alternatives. The suggestion from the nurse is that
there is a reason, but that he should not concern himself with it.

8. When caring for a client who is at risk from self-harm, the nurse can help in a variety of ways. She should establish an honest, friendly relationship where the person feels able to disclose his feelings without threat or loss of trust. In some situations of potential self-harm it may also be appropriate to work through the individual's perception of himself, those around him and his life situation. The latter response is not one which is normally favoured in a severe type of depression as deep analysis of self and others may only serve to increase feelings of hopelessness.

   Option B is the correct response.

   Options A, C and D: All suggest that fostering of self-understanding would be appropriate. As David's depressive reaction seems to be of a severe or retarded type this would not be appropriate.

9. It is not the responsibility of the nurse to prescribe medications. However, as she is in contact with the client for 24 hours, she is the most appropriate person to observe for unwanted effects of medications. A variety of reactions may occur in different people and the nurse must assume some responsibility for observing and recognising the major unwanted effects of chemotherapy. She should also be aware that initially most of the effects are likely to be presented in the form of complaints from the client as opposed to observable changes.

   Option D is the correct response.

   Options A, B and C: All contain the sensation of headaches. Whilst this may occur, it is certainly not a commonly encountered unwanted effect of tricyclic therapy.

Essay questions

1. David is a 48-year-old married man who has recently been admitted to a psychiatric unit. Over the past 6 months he has gradually lost interest in most things in his life, finds difficulty in maintaining conversations, and has developed ideas that he is suffering from a physical illness.

   A Describe the factors which might indicate to the nurse that this client's confidence is diminished, and that he is experiencing a lowering of his self-concept, self-image.   30%

   B Describe ways in which the nursing team can help to reduce the following areas of difficulty in his life:
   (i) Loss of self-confidence.   35%
   (ii) Reduced self-worth.   35%

2. David has recently been admitted to hospital. He has little interest in any aspect of his life and has recently expressed ideas that he feels a burden to his family.
   Outline nursing plans for this client in response to the following problems:

   A Self-neglect.   35%
   B Excessive concern regarding his physical well-being.   30%
   C Potential self-harm.   35%

3. David is a married man who has recently been admitted to a psychiatric unit. Some of the problems he is experiencing are a loss of interest, sadness, a slowing of his thoughts and actions, and a belief that he may be physically ill.
   He has a caring family who are worried and perplexed by what has happened to him.

   A Describe how the nursing team can promote the involvement of the family in the care of this client.   50%

   B Describe the skills and qualities which the nurse should display when his family ask, 'What is wrong with him?'   50%

Specimen answer

1. A   The image we have of ourselves is projected in virtually everything we do in our lives. It is these everyday factors that must be observed and checked against previous standards which can be obtained from significant individuals in the life of the client.

David is likely to experience 'awkwardness' in social situations, feeling insecure and threatened by apparently innocuous events. This may lead to a withdrawal from social contacts. He may display a reluctance to attempt new activities and experiences, or to make decisions, the thoughts of failure being ever present in his mind.

Outward appearance is also an aspect of self-image, and the standard of dress and hygiene of the client will most probably be affected by his thoughts.

In addition to those aspects which can be observed, there may be actual statements made by the client which serve to indicate his self-perception: statements such as 'I can't do this', 'I don't know why people bother with me', or 'Why am I causing so much trouble to everyone?'

B (i) *Self-confidence*

It is important, in attempting to build David's self-confidence, that the skills of encouragement, persuasion and support, along with the qualities of understanding, patience and genuineness, are carefully combined to produce the best results.

In areas such as social interaction it is better to use a non-threatening relationship on a one-to-one basis. Then, judging the speed of development carefully, move in ever widening circles of social contact. The choice of companions is just as important, and it is preferable to include clients who appear to have something in common or a bond developing between them.

Achievement can also be used as a tool to enhance both confidence and self-worth with the client initially working alongside the nurse in small, carefully chosen tasks, making tea and coffee or contributing to the social organisation of the environment. An extension of these activities would lead to more structured choices. In these choices it is advantageous to use activities which are new to the client in the first instance. David has no past reference points with these activities and it is more difficult, therefore, for him to compare present with past performances. Such comparisons could be used to reinforce his perception of himself. Furthermore, it allows the nurse to focus on the progress David is making by using his achievements as a yardstick.

The involvement of the client in decision-making is another way of developing his self-confidence. These decisions, as with social interactions, must be graded in intensity so that they do not become destructive. Initially, the decisions may focus upon simple tasks such as the choice of clothing to be worn that day, the nurse already having narrowed the choice to two or three items of clothing which seem compatible. The task then for the client is to choose between two or three items only and not a full wardrobe. In all of these processes it is essential that when any progress is made it is recognised and pointed out to David in a manner which is not patronising.

B (ii) *Self-worth*

Much of the work already outlined will also affect the self-perception of the client. As an additional and specific technique, the nurse could use the processes of cognitive therapy, enlisting the aid of the family in this process. Cognitive therapy is based upon several broad themes: firstly, that the client will use all his experiences to support and reinforce his assumption of worthlessness, secondly, to encourage the client to consider possible alternative thoughts; and finally, to try out those alternatives and associated actions.

In this way the nurse will use every oppoprtunity to interrupt the destructive cycle of low self-opinion, assumed failure, absence of action and further lowering of self-opinion. If interruption of this process can be achieved, then the nurse can attempt to establish a more realistic self-perception.

Answer guides

2. A *Self-neglect*

'In all of the areas concerned, the client's normal patterns of behaviour must be considered and, following assessment, care implemented where necessary.

Hygiene:
— encourage to wash, bathe and attend to hair and mouth care
— in some circumstances it may be necessary for the nurse to assume responsibility for these actions
— improvements in David's self-perception is likely to produce a return to his normal standards of hygiene.

Appearance:
— encourage David to dress himself
— assist where necessary
— appropriate choice of clothing
— praise and reinforcement where appropriate
— improve self-perception.

Diet:
— ensure appropriate foods
— take account of the preferences of the client
— give small amounts, attractively presented
— consideration should be given to dining area, pleasant setting
— supplementary fluids may be required

— weekly weight checks
— assistance with eating may have to be considered.
Exercise:
— encourage and accompany, if necessary, on some exercise daily.
Bowel care:
— provide adequate roughage and fluid intake
— ensure daily exercise.
   In all of these areas psychological interventions may also prove useful. The nurse could employ such techniques as modelling or instructing.

B   *Agitation and concern regarding physical well-being*
Assessment of physical condition by nursing and medical staff to exclude the possibility of organic disease. Do not deny the feelings of the client as they are real to him.
Do not agree with his thoughts of physical illness as this will reinforce his ideas and, as he improves, will damage relationships which have been established.
Sympathetically offer an explanation of how these feelings may have developed.
Offer support by giving him your time and energy.
Use techniques of diversion and distraction where appropriate. Ensure that medications are taken as prescribed.

C   *Self-harm*
Explanation to David of the concerns of others regarding his safety: encourage his involvement in the care plan. Discuss with relatives and friends the importance of liaising with staff regarding requests for equipment or substances which may be harmful.
Minimise access to the means of self-harm:
— ensure that medications are taken
— safety and correct use of equipment
— inform other work people regarding the safe storage of equipment
— observations
— structured day, giving time for activities which may serve to distract or divert the thoughts of the client.
Reduce motivation for self-harm:
— give of self
— encourage verbalisation beyond initial statements
— facilitate examination of feelings.

3. A On a general level the following methods could prove beneficial:
       — Approach and attitude displayed by the team should be open and welcoming.
       — Questions from the family must be dealt with as promptly and honestly as possible.
       — Regular contact between the family and nursing team should be established.

— Inclusion of the family in David care conferences.

More specifically related to the strategies of care, the family should be included in the processes of:

— Assessment: In order to gain a complete picture, the views of the family must be sought and assistance obtained in areas of assessment which David may not be able to complete.

— Planning: Inclusion of the family in discussions regarding goals and priorities. The family may then feel comfortable about reinforcing the ideas of the plan to David on the occasions that he forgets. Opportunities can be offered to discuss their views regarding follow-up processes, facilities available, and those which might be required in their case.

— Implementation: Because they have been involved in other stages of this process the family will be able to offer support during the actual giving of care. Encouragement could be given for members of the family to include themselves in some of the activities concerned, or indeed in aspects of the care of the client, such as assistance at meal-times.

— Evaluation: As with assessment, to ensure a balanced view it is important to obtain the views of the family regarding progress made in defined areas of difficulty.

B *Skills.*

Organisational:

— arranging duties and activities so that time can be spent with the family

— ensure that the setting is conducive to a free exchange of views, e.g., in terms of privacy and seating arrangements.

Communication:

— verbal:

   pace at which information is given

   tone of voice

   language used.

— non-verbal:

   posture

   angle of seating

   expression

   proximity

   touch.

Interviewing: asking the right question at the appropriate time is essential for the nurse to clarify what the family already know and what they wish to know.

Counselling: certain counselling skills may be appropriate. If the family seem angry or upset, then skills which facilitate ventilation of these feelings would be required.

Qualities.
Openness: a friendly, warm attitude should be displayed.
Willingness to invest time.
Non-judgemental approach so that the family feel able to express their feelings without fear of recriminations, either verbal or non-verbal.
Empathy: a difficult area, but one which the nurse should strive to achieve.
Confidence: the family will not wish to be dealt with by a nurse who is vague and obviously uncertain of both herself and her information.
Recognising limits, and awareness of when and to whom referrals should be made.

10. Loss of contact with reality associated with elation

Mrs Linda Chezwoski has recently been admitted compulsorily to a mixed acute ward following a period of excited and bizarre behaviour. Linda is 38 years old, and a little overweight. She lives with her husband, Jan, in a small house on the fringes of a large city. According to Jan, Linda has always been full of life, enjoying social contacts and pursuits.

Approximately 2 weeks ago Linda's behaviour seemed to change. She started to clean the house, but left it unfinished to begin washing all the clothes, a task also left incomplete. The activities which she felt needed attention resulted in her neglecting her physical needs and it became difficult for Jan to convince her to rest or take adequate nourishment. During these expressions of his concern Linda became quite irritable and said that she felt great. 'This was just the time to do all the jobs which needed attention.'

Over this 2 week period her behaviour gradually became more bizarre and intrusive. It culminated in her knocking on the doors of her neighbours' houses at midnight, explaining that she wanted to start a keep-fit club in the street and now was as good a time as any to start.

On admission she was dressed in bright clothes and jewellery, had applied excessive make-up, and kept insisting that she was fine and asking everyone she met for a kiss. When asked where she was and why, she replied. 'I am in hospital, forced to come here by the neighbours who are jealous of my super-powers. Whilst I am here I don't mind organising keep-fit classes for everyone, nurses as well of course.'

Multiple choice questions

1. Which one of the following groups contains features which are all associated with the psychiatric condition of mania?
   A Physical neglect, disinhibited behaviour and purposeless activity.
   B Disinhibited behaviour, purposeless activity and increased sensitivity to stimuli.
   C Purposeless activity, increased sensitivity to stimuli and physical neglect.
   D Increased sensitivity to stimuli, physical neglect and disinhibited behaviour.

2. Which one of the following would be the most appropriate response of the nurse when Linda attempts to make a female patient with a hemiplegia walk without assistance?
   A Divert Linda's attention on to something else and ensure that the other patient is given assistance.
   B Ensure that the other patient is cared for and quietly but firmly tell Linda that she must not do such things.
   C Supervise Linda's actions but only intervene if the other patient seems in danger.
   D Explain to Linda the correct way of offering assistance to a person with hemiplegia.

3. Which one of the following groups contains elements which would all be useful when considering activities for Linda? The activities should:
   A expend energy, involve detailed work and be easily completed.
   B involve detailed work, be easily completed and reduce competition.
   C be easily completed, reduce competition and expend energy.
   D reduce competition, expend energy and involve detailed work.

4. Which one of the following groups of interventions would all be appropriate for the nurse to make if Linda's husband reports that he is worried about her writing cheques for large amounts of money?
   A Establish the validity of his concerns, explain that this is a common occurrence and advise him that he could inform the bank regarding the cheques.
   B Explain that this is a common occurrence, advise him that he could inform the bank regarding the cheques and ensure that, if correct, the cheque book is removed into safe keeping.
   C Advise him that he could inform the bank regarding the cheques, ensure that, if correct, the cheque book is removed into safe keeping and establish the validity of his concerns.
   D Ensure that, if correct, the cheque book is removed into safe keeping, establish the validity of his concerns and explain that this is a common occurrence.

5. Which one of the following groups contains features which are all unwanted effects of lithium therapy?
   A Hypotension, gastro-intestinal disturbance and fine tremor.
   B Gastro-intestinal disturbance, fine tremor and polydipsia.
   C Fine tremor, polydipsia and hypotension.
   D Polydipsia, hypotension and gastro-intestinal disturbance.

6. Which one of the following would be the most appropriate response for the nurse to make if Linda refuses to take her prescribed medication, arguing that she has never felt better and does not need it?
   A Tell Linda a 'white lie' about the medication in an attempt to persuade her to take it.
   B Crush the medication concerned and ensure that it is given in a disguised form.
   C Inform Linda that because of the importance of the medication she will have to be given an injection if necessary.
   D Demonstrate an understanding of her feelings and explain the need to continue with medication regularly.

7. Which one of the following groups contains elements which all appertain to section 5(4) of the Mental Health Act 1983?
   A The safety of the individual or others is considered to be at risk, the responsible consultant must be informed immediately and the hospital managers must be notified promptly.
   B The responsible consultant must be informed immediately, the hospital managers must be notified promptly and the patient must be seen by a doctor within the period of the order.
   C The hospital managers must be notified promptly, the individual must be seen by a doctor within the period of the order and the safety of the individual or others is considered to be at risk.
   D The individual must be seen by a doctor within the period of the order, the safety of the individual or others is considered to be at risk and the responsible consultant must be notified immediately.

8. Which one of the following groups contains nursing interventions which would all be appropriate when caring for Linda?
   A Reinforce reality, display a non-judgemental attitude and explain everything to Linda in detail.
   B Display a non-judgemental attitude, explain everything to Linda in detail and model calm responses.
   C Explain everything to Linda in detail, model calm responses and reinforce reality.
   D Model calm responses, reinforce reality and display a non-judgemental attitude.

9. Which one of the following groups contains initial responses which would all be appropriate if Linda informs the nurse in charge that she is going to make an official complaint about nurses eating food intended for patients?
   A Clarify her perceptions of the situation, offer explanations which support and reinforce reality and remind her that she retains the right of complaint.
   B Offer explanations which support and reinforce reality, remind her that she retains the right of complaint and attempt to re-direct her thinking onto more positive areas.
   C Remind her that she retains the right of complaint, attempt to re-direct her thinking onto more positive areas and clarify her perceptions of the situation.
   D Attempt to re-direct her thinking onto more positive areas, clarify her perceptions of the situation and offer explanations which support and reinforce reality.

Answer keys to MCQs

1. The psychiatric condition of mania is classified as a psychotic illness within the definitions outlined in the World Health Organization, International Classification of Diseases. As a psychotic illness, there is classically a loss of insight. Also apparent in mania is an increase in psychomotor activity.

   Option D is the correct response. Because of an increase in psychic activity or awareness, sensitivity to stimuli is increased and anything which impinges upon any of the senses will be responded to. Physical neglect is a common feature because the individual concerned is too pre-occupied to consider spending time on such matters. Disinhibited behaviour also occurs, with the person saying and doing whatever they feel without restriction by the processes of conscience.

   Options A, B and C: All contain the features of purposeless activity. Whilst the person experiencing a manic reaction will be overactive, it will be activity with a purpose rather than without. For example the patient may dash from one end of the ward to the other in order to be there to open a door for a member of staff or visitors.

2. One of the characteristics of a person suffering from mania is her belief in her own abilities and a feeling that whatever she believes and does will be all right. This can extend to situations which are potentially hazardous to the individual concerned or those around her.

   Option A is the correct response as care is being given to both patients. No attempt should be made to argue with or reprimand Linda, but constructive use is made of her distractability and sensitivity to stimuli. At the same time the patient with a hemiplegia is also being cared for as she may be feeling anxious and vulnerable through Linda's actions.

   Option B: Linda believes that whatever she does is right, and within her control. To adopt an approach which sounds reprimanding would only result in confrontation. It may be necessary for the nurse to explain to Linda the consequences of her behaviour, but this could be done after the initial situation has been resolved.

   Options C and D: would not be appropriate as they suggest that a patient who is obviously vulnerable would be left in the care of a patient who is overactive, thus creating a potentially dangerous situation.

3. The presenting features of Linda's problems include an exaggerated view of her own abilities, excessive energy, low tolerance to frustration and increased sensitivity to stimuli. When considering the choice of activities, therefore, the nurse should be attempting to prevent confrontations and difficulties.

Option C is the correct response as the activity should allow Linda the opportunity to expend some of her energy in a controlled situation. Such a strategy also recognises that her concentration span is limited and does not involve competition, thereby reducing frustration and potential confrontation.

Options A, B and D: All include the choice of detailed work. This type of activity would be inappropriate because of Linda's distractability, reduced concentration span and low tolerance to frustration.

4. Exaggerated ideas regarding abilities, status and wealth are common features of the condition of mania. To safeguard patients and their families from abuse as a result of these beliefs, it is normal practice to ensure the removal into safe-keeping of items such as cheque books, credit cards and cash. However, even the most vigilant nurse may find that a patient has managed to obtain such items, perhaps from relatives who do not appreciate the consequences of their actions.

Option C is the correct response. The first action of the nurse should be to listen to Linda's husband and determine the source of evidence for his concerns. If it is established that Linda still has access to a cheque book this should be removed into safe-keeping. Should Linda's husband still be concerned, he could be advised regarding other courses of action such as informing his bank to stop the cheques.

Options A, B and D: All suggest that the nurse could explain to Linda's husband that this was a common occurrence. This response would not help him as his anxieties are real and are focussed only on what is happening now. Positive action from the nurse will reassure him more than statements which are only intended to pacify.

5. Lithium salts are not a naturally occurring bodily substance. It has been found that if lithium salts are administered to obtain controlled serum levels they can be an effective remedial therapy for states of mania or they can be used as a prophylactic measure in manic-depressive conditions.

Dosage and serum lithium levels are closely monitored, the aim being to produce a serum concentration of 0.6–1.2 mmol/litre.

When administering lithium it is important for the nurse to remember that certain preparations act on a slow-release basis and as such must not be crushed.

Option B is the correct response. The common unwanted effects of lithium therapy are anorexia, nausea, diarrhoea, polyuria, polydipsia, fine tremor and ataxia.

Options A, C and D: All include hypotension which although a problem with many drugs has not been recorded as a significant problem with patients on lithium therapy.

6. As Linda has never felt better, this type of response is one to be expected. Occasionally, other manifestations of the same feelings occur, such as wishing to leave the hospital, not needing food or rest and attempting impossible tasks.
   The response of the nurse should be non-threatening and not destructive to relationships which have been established.

   Option D is the correct response as it presents a mature and open statement by the nurse. If such a response is ineffective then other strategies may have to be considered; each one, however, should seek to maintain the dignity of the individual and be honest in its content.

   Option A: This type of response may on occasions be successful in persuading a patient to take medications, but as the person recovers, such techniques will be remembered and the maintenance of the nurse–patient relationship will become more difficult.

   Option B: Priadel® is one of the preparations of lithium which should not be crushed. This aspect alone renders the response inappropriate; in addition to which it is better to be honest and not surreptitious when giving medications to patients.

   Option C: Although it is possible that the medication may have to be administered by another route this cannot be certain until it has been checked with the responsible medical officer. Another aspect is that the response should not appear threatening as this is only likely to provoke an aggressive display.

7. Section 5(4) of the Mental Health Act 1983 refers to the nurse's holding power. Under this section a nurse of the prescribed class—Registered—may detain a patient when the safety of the patient or others is considered to be at risk. Within the period of detention the patient must be seen by a doctor. It is the responsibility of the nurse to complete the necessary documentation and inform the hospital managers as soon as possible.

   Option C is the correct response.

   Options A, B and D: All include the need to inform the responsible consultant immediately. Whilst it is a requirement that the patient be seen by a doctor within the specified time, it is not stipulated that this should be a consultant.

8. The interventions and actions of the nurse should have regard for Linda's overactivity, loss of contact with reality and uninhibited behaviour.

Option D is the correct response. The nurse should display calmness in general actions and also in responding to specific situations. It is impossible to resolve the problem of loss of insight in the short term; however, the nurse can present to Linda an image of reality as she sees it. This would be an honest reaction and the consistency required in such a response would not interfere with the development or maintenance of therapeutic relationships. Some of Linda's observations and actions will not be governed by social conventions and may disturb those around her. The nurse should present firm but non-threatening guidelines of acceptable behaviours, but at the same time display an attitude which is not shocked or judgemental.

Options A, B and C: It is of course the right of every patient to know what is planned in her care and treatment. However, because of Linda's limited concentration span and degree of distractability it would most probably be counter-productive to try to explain everything in great detail.

9. As Linda responds quickly to stimuli and is uninhibited in her actions, accusations of this type are regular occurrences. In many instances the complaints are based upon inaccurate perceptions and a loss of contact with reality. Because many such complaints are mistakes, it is very easy for the nurse to dismiss all allegations as inaccurate.

Option A is the correct response. The nurse must acknowledge that all such complaints may be accurate and investigate thoroughly, commencing with the patient's view of the circumstances and events. If the nurse believes, after investigation, that the report is inaccurate she should attempt to reinforce reality by explaining the situation as she sees it. Reinforcement of this nature may prove ineffective. If this is the case, the individual concerned retains the right to register her complaint to other personnel such as the senior nurse manager.

Options B, C and D: All suggest that Linda's thoughts should be directed onto more positive areas. This may be a useful strategy later in the proceedings but not as an initial response. To take such action would indicate that the nurse believed the accusation to be false and this cannot be certain before investigation.

Essay questions

1. Linda Chezwoski has recently been admitted to a mixed acute unit. On admission she was overactive and disinhibited; she dressed brightly, was ultra-sensitive to stimuli and expressed an exaggerated opinion of her abilities.

   A What factors may interfere with communication processes between Linda and the nursing staff?   25%

   B Describe ways in which the nursing staff could attempt to overcome the difficulties of communicating with this client.   50%

   C Describe the environmental factors of the ward which should be considered when caring for Linda.   25%

2. Linda is a 38-year-old married woman who has been admitted to a mixed acute ward. She is displaying behaviour associated with elation and overactivity.

   Describe interventions which the nurse could use in response to the following problems, identified during the process of assessment.

   A High level of distractability—limited concentration span.   35%

   B Overactivity—difficulty in taking adequate rest.   30%

   C Physical neglect related particularly to hygiene and nutrition.   35%

3. Linda is a married woman who has been displaying signs of overactivity, personal neglect, and disinhibited behaviour.

   A Describe nursing interventions that could be made in response to Linda repeatedly making sexual suggestions and advances towards a number of male patients on the ward.   35%

   B What could be the nurse's response, and why, when Linda's husband complains that he feels his wife is at risk on a mixed ward and would prefer her to be moved to another ward?   30%

   C Explain how the nurse in charge can help a recently allocated and relatively inexperienced nurse who states that she is frustrated and irritable when caring for this client.   35%

Specimen answer

1. A The overactivity which Linda is displaying, and her beliefs that there are many important tasks for her to do, will relegate communication to a position of secondary importance. She is also very sensitive to stimuli and among the ways in which this will present is difficulty in concentrating on a specific subject or task, e.g. constantly changing from one topic to another.

   Associated with these rapid thought processes is a speech pattern which is much quicker than normal: the words may tumble out at such speed that the nurse finds it difficult to comprehend what is being said. Disinhibited thinking is likely to interfere with interpersonal communication due to the inclusion in conversations of anything that Linda feels like saying.

   Another aspect of Linda's perceptions which may disrupt normal communication is her belief in her own abilities and importance. The nurse may be summarily dismissed by Linda when the interaction does not seem to have any more importance.

   In addition, the nurse's attitudes towards Linda, her past experience and the demands upon her time may also disrupt the process of communication.

   B In examining ways in which the process of communication can be enhanced, the nurse must give consideration to those factors which are thought to interfere with communication.

   When responding to overactivity the nurse must be prepared for communication to occur through repeated contacts of short duration which take account of Linda's limited concentration span. Another strategy which could be used by the nurse is working alongside Linda. Through working together the nurse could encourage her to rest, and should herself model calm responses.

   If Linda suggests that the subject concerned is unimportant, or that she is above this type of concern, the nurse should maintain a calm and consistent approach. She should try not to increase Linda's frustration by arguing, but rather she should attempt to explain the situation clearly and in this way reinforce reality.

   When Linda speaks very quickly the nurse should encourage her to slow down, perhaps by modelling an appropriate type of speech. Key words may also be identified in what Linda is saying and used as a basis for communication. If in doubt the nurse could ask Linda to explain what she has said. The nurse should be aware that correcting or inhibiting the patient can lead to irritability and frustration.

   Because of Linda's sensitivity to stimuli the nurse should speak slowly but not in a condescending manner, using key words or short questions as a means of asking, suggesting or persuading. It is also possible, if other methods fail, to convey some information in writing, using the same principles which apply to verbal communication.

   Overall, the nurse should display a non-judgemental approach to Linda's behaviour, and persuade her to focus on here-and-now issues.

C Reducing stimuli and preventing accidents must be the main considerations
when planning the environment in which Linda is to be nursed.

Measures which help to reduce stimuli are those of reducing noise levels
as much as possible and ensuring that lighting is not glaring or intrusive,
providing a decor which is relaxing and avoiding extremes of temperature.

In an attempt to prevent accidents care should be taken with equipment
and floor surfaces. Explanations could also be given to visiting workmen
regarding the importance of keeping tools and equipment safe. These
aspects apply equally to any patient in hospital; however, Linda's vulnerbility
to accidents is increased because of her presenting symptoms.

Answer guides

2. A *Distractability—limited concentration span*
   Verbal responses:
   — level, tone, and controlled volume of voice
   — restricted speed of conversation
   — content should be simple questions or statements
   — focussing.
   Non-verbal responses:
   — attitude should be:
     tolerant
     calm, controlled
     non-judgemental
   — nurse's awareness of own gestures and mannerisms.
   Reduction of stimuli:
   — noise levels
   — lighting
   — decor
   — degree of activity in clinical area
   — temperature control
   — limit number of different staff involved in interventions.
   Choice of activities:
   — easily completed
   — short in duration
   — avoid intricate work
   — encourage perseverance.
   Positive aspects of distractability:
   — persuasion
   — re-direction
   — ensure frequent contacts of short duration.
 B *Overactivity—inability to rest*
   Channel energy:
   — useful exercise in a controlled situation.

Encourage rest:
— company
— conversation
— explanations.
Relaxation strategies:
— tone of voice
— warm drinks
— warm baths
— reduce stimuli
— music.
Ensure safety:
— floor coverings
— equipment
— clothing.
Chemotherapy:
— ensure medications are taken as prescribed.

C *Physical neglect—nutrition*
Encouragement:
— explanation of nutritional needs
— conducive situations, i.e., dining area
— sit down with the patient
— determine likes and dislikes
— small portions given often: care must be taken regarding the risk of choking, as Linda may be inclined to rush her food.
Alternative strategies:
— 'mobile foods', e.g., sandwiches, boiled eggs (shelled), pieces of cheese, fruit (peeled if necessary)
— supplementary fluids
— liquidised meals.
Fluids:
— dehydration is a risk because of lack of time to drink combined with overactivity and perspiration
— careful control of temperature of drinks is required as they are likely to be rushed.

Physical neglect—hygiene
Encouragement:
— explanation of hygiene/health
— use of persuasion, suggestion.
Bathing:
— because of perspiration and neglected toilet hygiene.
Sanitary needs:
— encouragement
— explanation

— responsibility may have to be taken by the nurse
— modelling general standards of hygiene.

3. A *Approach and attitude:*
— acceptance
— tolerance
— non-judgemental
— understanding the feelings of everyone involved
— consistency.
Observation:
— ensure Linda's well-being and protection.
Explanation:
— give to Linda a firm but fair explanation of the effects of her behaviour on others
— give to others, whilst retaining the principle of confidentiality as far as possible, a clear and concise account of such behaviour and possible strategies to adopt in response.
Diversion:
— ensure a planned programme of care
— distract if possible in immediate situation.
B *Acceptance of concerns:*
— make time for discussion
— organise setting to be as conducive as possible.
Clarify:
— his perceptions of the situation
— his feelings.
Explanations:
— of Linda's behaviour
— of facilities, i.e., separation of male and female patients
— observations of nurses as a means of protection.
Cathartic ventilation:
— appropriate questions
— encourage ventilation of feelings
— understanding of his feelings.
Openness:
— explanation of and access to alternative personnel who can be consulted, i.e., nursing or medical staff.
Reviews:
— remain open to further expressions of concern
— make positive efforts to re-assess his feelings at a later time.

C *Exploration of the reason for these feelings:*
— the nurse's view of Linda
— preconceived ideas
— anxiety or fear
— feelings of skill inadequacy
— the nurse's concept of the patient role.
Prevent feelings of isolation:
— acceptance of feelings
— explanation regarding difficulties experienced by many nurses when responding to such behaviours.
Encourage the nurse's acceptance of Linda:
— explanation of Linda's perceptions
— consider involving other personnel, e.g., teaching staff or nurse managers.
Promote feelings of involvement:
— explanation of care plan
— discussion of specific responses and strategies.
Assist with skill development:
— explore techniques or interventions which may be effective when responding to Linda's behaviours and statements
— discuss importance of not letting feelings become apparent to Linda
— careful assessment of delegated responsibilities.
Evaluation:
— review the feelings of the nurse on a pre-arranged date
— feedback to the nurse the views of senior nurses.

11. Loss of contact with reality associated with disintegrative thought processes

Quentin Chapman is 22 years old, the youngest of four children raised in the problem area of a council estate. At school he initially did well, though he was often teased for his dirty dishevelled appearance. His school reports made consistent remarks about his lack of concentration and his ability to perform better. Since leaving school he has had numerous jobs in packing, portering and light assembly work.

Six months ago he began to develop ideas that the Special Branch were watching him and keeping a dossier on his activities. One month ago he was admitted to hospital after an impulsive attack on a man in the street whom he believed to be tracking his movements with a 'pedograph'. Since that time he has been largely uncommunicative and answers questions in monosyllables. He will not mix with other patients and prefers to eat alone. On occasions he can be seen sitting rocking in the chair smiling and grimacing for no apparent reason. Sometimes he can be heard in isolated parts of the ward shouting unintelligible statements. In the ward he wears a flat cap and a large overcoat with the collar turned up to his ears. His trousers are tied at the bottom with string and on his feet he wears open-toed sandals. He neglects his physical hygiene and often appears unwashed, unkempt and unshaven.

Multiple choice questions

1. Which one of the following would be the best response if Quentin states: 'The Special Branch are all around, they want me dead'?
   A 'It must be very frightening for you to feel that way; however, I see no indication that they are here'.
   B 'Don't worry about that, I'm sure no one wants to hurt you.'
   C 'The Special Branch deal with items of national security; where is your evidence that they are interested in you?'
   D 'Try not to worry about it. Would you like to watch television'.

2. Which one of the following groups contains interventions which would help to reverse the patient's withdrawn behaviour in the early stages of his care?
   A Make contact on a one-to-one basis, respect need for personal space and involve in group discussion.
   B Respect need for personal space, increase eye-to-eye contact and involve in group discussion.
   C Make contact on a one-to-one basis, involve in group discussion and increase eye-to-eye contact.
   D Respect need for personal space, make contact on a one-to-one basis and increase eye-to-eye contact.

3. Which one of the following actions will help to reduce Quentin's misunderstandings of nursing interventions?
   A Make physical contact, minimise non-verbal communication and avoid metaphors and complex sentences.
   B Speak clearly and concretely, minimise non-verbal messages and avoid metaphors and complex sentences.
   C Avoid metaphors and complex sentences, speak clearly and concretely and make physical contact.
   D Make physical contact, speak clearly and concretely and minimise non-verbal messages.

4. Which one of the following statements best describes the reason why nurses should state their own beliefs simply and calmly when patients express delusions?
   That it:
   A provides an alternative frame of reference whilst validating reality.
   B demonstrates to the patient that the nurse has a genuine interest in his beliefs.
   C provides the means and opportunity whereby the patient's ideas can be logically discussed.
   D encourages the patient to further elaborate his thoughts and feelings.

5. Which one of the following groups of symptoms would help to confirm a diagnosis of a schizophrenic disorder?
   A Ideas that thoughts are being inserted into the mind, that voices are giving a running commentary of the person's behaviour and that real perceptions are mistakenly interpreted.
   B That experiences are imposed on the person against their will, real perceptions are mistakenly interpreted and ideas that thoughts are being inserted into the mind.
   C That real perceptions are mistakenly interpreted, that voices are giving a running commentary of the person's behaviour and that experiences are imposed on the person against their will.
   D That voices are giving a running commentary of the person's behaviour, that experiences are imposed on the person against their will and that thoughts are being inserted into the mind.

6. Which one of the following interventions would best help Quentin to develop a more appropriate style of dress and appearance?
   A Offer tokens, which can be exchanged for rewards, for appropriate dress and appearance.
   B Involve in unstructured group work as a means of increasing self-awareness.
   C Give negative or positive feedback contingent upon dress and appearance.
   D Put out appropriate clothing and ensure reasonable dress and hygiene.

7. Which one of the following groups contains factors, identified in Quentin's background, which have been associated with an increased expectation of the development of a schizophrenic disorder?
   A Background in social class V, the youngest of a large sibling group and solitariness in childhood and adolescence.
   B Solitariness in childhood and adolescence, failure to live up to early expectations and a background in social class V.
   C Failure to live up to early expectations, a background in social class V and the youngest in a large sibling group.
   D Failure to live up to early expectations, the youngest in a large sibling group and solitariness in childhood and adolescence.

8. Which one of the following groups contains interventions which would be of value, in the early stages of Quentin's care, in response to his rocking, smiling and grimacing?
   A Provide a structured day, involve the full ward community in his programme and give concrete physical tasks to perform.
   B Involve the full ward community in his programme, give concrete physical tasks to perform and gradually increase personal contact.
   C Give concrete physical tasks to perform, gradually increase personal contact and provide a structured day.
   D Gradually increase personal contact, provide a structured day and involve the full ward community in his programme.

9. Which one of the following criteria would suggest a favourable prognosis for Quentin.
   A Acute onset of symptoms.
   B Emotional blunting.
   C Evidence of first rank symptoms.
   D No obvious precipitating cause.

Answer keys to MCQs

1. A number of principles determines the most appropriate response to delusional speech. The main one includes accepting the person whilst taking care not to argue with or to validate the delusional ideas.

   Option A is the correct response. It recognises Quentin as a person and would thus help to build up a trusting relationship. It recognises the patient's feelings which are real and empathises with them. The reply neither argues with nor validates Quentin's perception but is nevertheless based on reality and provides an alternative frame of reference regarding his ideas.

   Option B fails to recognise Quentin's feelings and tends to minimise his distress.

   Option C attempts to deal with the statement by the application of logic when such statements are inaccessible to that type of intervention.

   Option D is an attempt to distract and thus change the subject which may be desirable but fails to recognise the patient's feelings and may lead to an unwillingness to share information in the future.

2. Withdrawal frequently occurs as a defence against interpersonal stress. Intensity in relationships should be avoided. The approach should be non-threatening and others should only be introduced on a gradual basis.

   Option D is the correct response. All of the interventions would be appropriate. Where people are out of contact with reality and feel that others are planning to hurt them, then the need to respect personal space must be adhered to. If this is not done, then the approach may be seen as threatening and may increase withdrawal or alternatively provoke an aggressive response. It is essential that contact is made initially on a one-to-one basis and that trust develops before introducing others into the regime. It is important to pay attention to non-verbal communication, such as eye contact, approaching from front and use of non-threatening postures, when working with such clients. Eye contact should be gradually increased as a way of making contact and building up trust.

   Options A, B and C: All contain involvement with groups of people which should come later into a plan of care. Additionally group discussion tends to revolve around thoughts, ideas, concepts, attitudes and feelings, whilst the need is for more structure in the initial stages with activities of a physical concrete nature, firmly based in reality.

3. Misinterpretation of actions and communications frequently transpire in atmospheres and situations of mistrust. Clients who are both suspicious and out of touch with reality may well mistake a nurse's behaviour as some form of attack or plot if care is not taken.

Option B is the correct response. All of the actions would be appropriate. The verbal statements should be given clearly and concretely to avoid half-heard messages which could be misinterpreted. Speaking concretely bases the statements in reality. Metaphors, similes and complex sentences should be avoided due to the client's tendency to concrete thinking and lowered span of concentration. There is a risk of non-verbal communications being misunderstood as signals or threatening gestures. Attention and awareness should be developed in this area.

Options A, C and D: contain the action of making physical contact. This can easily be seen as threatening. Such clients have difficulty in maintaining self-concept and personal boundaries, and may find physical contact frightening and intrusive.

4. One of the principles of responding to a patient's delusional speech is that the practitioner should clearly and calmly offer his or her own beliefs about the idea under discussion.

Option A is the correct response. This gives feedback to the patient about the nurse's perception without stepping into the patient's world. It demonstrates that the nurse is listening without reinforcing the delusional statement. The response should be delivered simply and calmly to avoid misinterpretation and challenge.

Option B concentrates on the mistaken beliefs and will tend to reinforce these.

Option C suggests that individuals experiencing delusional thinking are accessible to debate, question or logic which they are not.

Option D will reinforce by positive encouragement the expression of delusional material.

5. A diagnosis of schizophrenia is more likely when a number of symptoms are found together. Some symptoms are found in many different conditions whilst others occur principally in schizophrenic disorders and are termed first rank symptoms. This classification was originally formulated by a psychiatrist named Schneider and for that reason the symptoms are sometimes referred to as 'Schneider's first rank symptoms of schizophrenia'.

Option D is the correct response. All of the symptoms would help to confirm a diagnosis of schizophrenia. The question relates to first rank symptoms of schizophrenia which include:

Passivity experiences
— made experiences
— thought insertion
— thought withdrawal
— thought broadcasting
Hallucinations
— running commentary
— discussing in the third person
— audible thoughts
Primary delusions.

Options A, B and C: All contain 'a perception mistakenly interpreted.' This is a definition of an illusion. This is not a first rank symptom and occurs in many psychiatric and non-psychiatric situations.

6. Inappropriate and bizarre dress may be used by someone out of touch with reality as an expression of his inner thought disorder. Whilst standards of dress and appearance are considerations for the individual to make, nevertheless strange and bizarre apparel does have impact on others and may make it more difficult for the individual to receive society's acceptance.

Option C is the correct response. This provides a realistic framework within which the person can understand better his impact on others. The feedback should be given clearly and directly and be directed to behaviour which the person can do something about rather than personal qualities which they may not. Negative feedback does not imply criticism but rather a constructive opinion which is offered in such a way that the person is left free to accept or reject it.

Option A is more appropriate in a context of working with dependent and institutionalised patients.

Option B would tend to be too threatening for Quentin and he would be unlikely to gain from it. People who have psychiatric disorders have difficulty in relating to abstract thoughts and ideas. They may find intimacy, particularly where large numbers are concerned, intimidating and destructive and are likely to move further into fantasy.

Option D takes too much responsibility away from the person and invests it in the nurse. The patient may be neat and tidy but this would be a reflection of the nurse's value system rather than the patient's. Dependency would be encouraged by this style of intervention.

7. A number of studies have identified factors which are associated with an increased expectation of schizophrenia. None of these studies is conclusive, and the factors are not causes though they do provide some indications.

Option B is the correct response. All the factors have been associated with the development of schizophrenia. Solitariness in childhood and adolescence is often retrospectively commented upon by parents and teachers and may indicate that withdrawal is being used as a coping strategy for interpersonal difficulties. A failure to live up to early expectations may also be noted. This may be due to concentration difficulties or problems with concepts and ideas and the development of abstract thinking. There is an increased incidence of schizophrenia evident in social class V and whilst environmental arguments have been put forward to explain this it does not alter the demographic fact.

Options A, C and D: contain the youngest of a large sibling group. This has no association with the development of schizophrenia.

8. Solitary rocking with smiling and grimacing are descriptive of autistic behaviour or extreme withdrawal. This is often a response to real or perceived threat and the management must take account of that whilst trying to provide worthwhile activity.

Option C is the correct response. All of the interventions would be of value. The principles of management are to provide structure and purpose to the day with tasks firmly based in reality, whilst recognising that withdrawal and autistic behaviour are responses to real or perceived threat. Interpersonal contact should be increased gradually, and only later should others be introduced into the programme when anxiety has been reduced and personal boundaries are secure.

Options A, B and D: All contain involving the full ward community in his programme. Withdrawal occurs as a response to feelings of insecurity and fear. Involving others in Quentin's programme would be likely to exacerbate these fears and lead to further withdrawal.

9. Prognosis and level of recovery vary with the individual but do tend to be linked to certain factors associated with the situation prior to breakdown and the features present at breakdown.

Option A is the correct response based upon the following prognostic criteria:

Good	Poor
No family history	Other members affected
Stable personality	Solitary and eccentric
Warm, stable relationships	Poverty of relationships
Stable home life	Stormy family relationships
Triggering life event	No obvious event
Acute onset	Insidious onset
Few first rank symptoms	Many first rank symptoms
Emotional response	Emotional blunting

Options B, C and D: All contain criteria which are indicative of a poor prognosis as shown in the above table.

Essay questions

1. Quentin Chapman, aged 22 years, has recently developed ideas that the Special Branch are keeping him under serveillance and tracking his every movement. In the ward he wears a flat cap and an overcoat with the collar turned up to his ears. His trousers are tied at the bottom with string and he wears open-toed sandals. He neglects his physical appearance and often appears unwashed, unkempt and unshaven.

   A How may Quentin be helped to develop a more appropriate dress and appearance?   50%

   B Give an appropriate verbal response of the nurse to Quentin's statement: 'The special branch are all around, they want me dead'.   20%

   C Discuss the therapeutic value of the response made.   30%

2. Quentin Chapman is a young man on an acute admission ward. He tends to be isolated and withdrawn and does not mix with others on the ward. He sits alone rocking in the chair, smiling and grimacing, and answers only when spoken to. On occasions he can be heard, in isolated parts of the ward, shouting unintelligible remarks.

   A What are the possible reasons underlying this behaviour?   20%

   B Describe a plan of nursing care which may improve Quentin's social interaction.   40%

   C Describe nursing interventions in response to his shouting.   40%

3. Quentin Chapman is 22 years of age and is admitted to the ward following an unprovoked attack on a man in the street. He states that the Special Branch has him under serveillance and that the man was 'Kertracking his mombulants with a pedograph'.

   A Describe the most likely reason for this form of speech.   15%

   B Describe how the nurse should respond to this form of speech giving reasons for the responses.   35%

   C Describe a plan of nursing care which would increase Quentin's contact with reality.   50%

Specimen answer

1. A The interventions will revolve around role modelling, teaching, feedback and positive reinforcement. For these to be effective the nurse needs to build up a relationship based upon trust and mutual respect so that the client will value the nurse's contribution. The nurse could act as an appropriate role model for the patient and demonstrate in her own dress and appearance a model which allows for the expression of individuality whilst maintaining an environmental and social awareness. Contact with reality should be encouraged as it is possible that the patient's appearance is a response to disordered thinking, e.g., delusional, or perceptual disturbance. The nurse should give realistic feedback to the patient based on the principles outlined in the following paragraph.

   The focus should be on behaviour not the person; the statement should be clear, direct and given with the object of building up rather than diminishing the person's self-concept. Appropriate dress and appearance should be positively reinforced by recognition and acknowledgement. Involvement in social skills training groups may reinforce the teaching, practice and feedback. Nurses should be careful not to impose their own values and should discourage staff, other patients and visitors from ridiculing or scorning the patient.

   B The response should be one that accepts the feeling but not the content of the statement. It should concentrate on reality without arguing with or validating delusional material, e.g., 'That must be very frightening for you. There are a lot of people here that you don't know but I don't believe that any wish to harm you'.

   C This response, most importantly, recognises the person's feelings of fear and apprehension and thereby helps in maintaining an effective working relationship. The feelings of the patient are real and it is, therefore, reasonable to respond to them. The content of Quentin's statement is not based in reality and should be neither argued with nor validated. The statement makes links between the feelings, the patient's conception and the reality of the situation. The nurse's own view of the situation is given calmly and clearly which allows the patient to appreciate an alternative frame of reference.

Answer guides

2. A Behaviour is likely to be a result of psychotic disorder:
   — sitting alone and rocking is autistic behaviour.
   — smiling and grimacing may be due to hallucinations.
   — environmental circumstances will also play a part.

   B Assessment and behavioural analysis and formation of base-lines. Contact on a one-to-one basis; adopt non-threatening postures and approach; presence may be sufficient initially.

Gradual increase of non-verbal contact.
Move to verbal communication; avoid interrogative communication.
Reward any speech or other interpersonal contact and particularly patient-initiated conversation.
Introduce others slowly; provide activities which offer relatedness without threat, i.e., walks, games.
Involve in situations and pastimes which stimulate.
Encourage involvement with family and contacts outside hospital. Increase social contact in and out of hospital.

C Behavioural analysis of:
— antecedants
— behaviour
— consequences.
Modify any factors stimulating or rewarding the behaviour.
Consistent approach, elements of limit-setting.
Model appropriate acceptable behaviour.
Involve in non-hospital settings.
Confront 'mad' behaviour.
Provide structure and purpose to the day.

3. A Speech contains neologisms used to describe bizarre experiences:
— evidence of thought disorder
— need to check that words are not dialect or malapropisms.

B Statement should be accepted as a genuine attempt at communication.
— Don't laugh or ridicule or in other ways discount the person.
— State inability to understand and seek to further communicate by using commonly accepted expressions.
— Model clear and direct speech.
— Don't use the neologisms.
— Give time and opportunity for client to clarify his statements.

C Recognise that fear and anxiety, especially concerned with interpersonal contact, will be present.
— Work on developing a trusting, accepting relationship.
— Care with non-verbal gestures.
— Non-verbal communication should mirror and be consistent with verbal.
— Accept feelings behind delusional speech not the content.
— Offer own perspectives as an alternative frame of reference.
— Engage in activities which are concrete and based in reality.
— Avoid games, activities which involve fantasy.
— Avoid role play, psychodrama as these tend to make real that which is not.
— Gradually introduce others into the situation.

12. The experience of continuing care and its effects

Dunstan Ward houses a group of male and female patients who have been in hospital for a number of years. In the past there have been few active treatment programmes and many of the patients are described as institutionalised.

Recently, there have been changes in the organisation of wards and programmes within the hospital. It is now planned to offer a more active rehabilitation structure. The abilities of the patients on the ward varies quite widely, though all have some degree of behavioural handicap or deficiency.

Multiple choice questions

1. Which one of the following groups contains organisations which could all be described as total institutions?
   A Convents, boarding schools and the police force.
   B The police force, the armed forces and government departments.
   C Government departments, the armed forces and boarding schools.
   D Boarding schools, the armed forces and convents.

2. Which one of the following groups contains features which are all descriptive of the total institution?
   A Changes in the work/payment structure, the presence of admission rituals and all life is carried out in the same place.
   B The presence of admission rituals, all life is carried out in the same place and a merging of staff and resident worlds.
   C All life is carried out in the same place, a merging of staff and resident worlds and changes in the work/payment structure.
   D A merging of staff and resident worlds, changes in the work/payment structure and the presence of admission rituals.

3. Which one of the following groups contains factors which have all been identified as responsible for the process of institutionalisation?
   A Hierachical staff structures, fixed meal and work times and enforced idleness.
   B Fixed meal and work times, enforced idleness and excessive use of tranquillising drugs.
   C Enforced idleness, excessive use of tranquillising drugs and hierarchical staff structures.
   D Excessive use of tranquillising drugs, hierarchical staff structures and fixed meal and work times.

4. Which one of the following groups contains descriptions which could all be applied to the institutionalised patient?
   A Resentment of harsh orders, withdrawal from others and a failure to plan for the future.
   B Withdrawal from others, a failure to plan for the future and a lack of motivation.
   C A failure to plan for the future, a lack of motivation and resentment of harsh orders.
   D A lack of motivation, resentment of harsh orders and withdrawal from others.

5. Which one of the following groups contains features which all provide a rationale for making base-line measurements of behaviour?
   A To discover the full range of problem behaviours, to target the most important handicaps and deficiencies, and to analyse the antecedents and consequences of specific behaviours.
   B To target the most important handicaps and deficiencies, to analyse the antecedents and consequences of specific behaviours and to enable judgements to be made on the effectiveness of treatment programmes.
   C To target the most important handicaps and deficiencies, to enable judgements to be made on the effectiveness of treatment programmes and to discover the full range of problem behaviours.
   D To analyse the antecedents and consequences of specific behaviours, to discover the full range of problem behaviours and to enable judgements to be made on the effectiveness of treatment programmes.

6. Which one of the following could be classed as an antecedent of a patient's stamping and shouting, observed as part of a behavioural analysis?
   A Sitting alone in a corner of the room.
   B Past experience of bizarre behaviours from other patients.
   C Isolation from general social norms.
   D Lowered performance expectations.

7. Which one of the following features should apply to a schedule of reinforcement as part of a behaviour modification programme? That rewards should:
   A be applied to all patients equally.
   B consist of physical, tangible goods or tokens.
   C remain unchanged for given behaviours.
   D be given as close to the behaviour as possible.

8. Which one of the following provides a description of shaping as a technique for modifying behaviour?
   A Demonstrating behavioural sequences and rewarding subsequent attempts.
   B Reinforcing behaviour which successively approximates to the desired outcomes.
   C Giving hints and reminders for behaviour and reinforcing subsequent attempts.
   D Gradually removing prompts to behaviour and rewarding activities undertaken through initiative.

9. Which one of the following groups contains components which would all form part of a social skills training programme?
   A Looking after hygiene and grooming, making requests of others and offering greetings and goodbyes.
   B Making requests of others, offering greetings and goodbyes and making eye contact.
   C Offering greetings and goodbyes, making eye contact and looking after hygiene and grooming.
   D Making eye contact, looking after hygiene and grooming and making requests of others.

Answer keys to MCQs

1. A total institution has been defined as one in which all life is carried out by the same people in the same place. Such features are apparent in organisations other than mental hospitals.

   Option D is the correct response. All of the organisations may be clasified as total institutions. One of the major factors is the 24 hour nature of the service or organisational structure. By necessity such institutions become removed from normal social routines and the more extreme the organisation the more pervasive the isolation.

   Options A, B and C: contain either the police force or government departments. Such organisations may have rigid structures, hierarchical management and profound bureaucracy but do not cover the total life experience of their members.

2. The total institution has many characteristics which distinguish it from other forms of organisation.

   Option A is the correct response. All of the features are descriptive of the total institution.

   A change in the work/payment structure is one of the main features. Members are required to work long hours often in mundane or unpleasant work for little reward. This is less often seen in psychiatric hospitals than was formerly the case, where patients had to maintain the basic amenities such as cleaning and laundering. However, some 'ward workers' still remain, carrying out duties from early morning to late evening, seven days a week, often for a pittance. Sometimes patients can be taken advantage of under the name of 'therapy'.

   Admission rituals serve to symbolically represent the giving up of past roles and responsibilities and the taking up of the roles of the institution. Some organisations have elaborate admission rituals which signify the total acceptance of the organisation and its philosophy. These rites of passage form part of the social stripping process which prepares the individual for his new life.

   The more of life that is carried out in the institution, the more extreme or total it becomes. Prisons are examples of extreme organisations. Psychiatric hospitals are making attempts to maintain links with communities and thus become less isolated and extreme.

   Options B, C and D: All include a merging of the staff and residents' worlds. The true nature of the relationship is of a split between staff and resident related to forms of address, permitted activities and social talk. Eating, toileting, sleeping and other activities are engaged in separately and distinctly with reserved sites and times for the differing groups.

3. There are many factors which lead to institutionalisation and dependency, particularly in wards for long-stay patients in psychiatric hospitals.

Option C is the correct response. All of the factors indicated may lead to institutionalisation.

There is a profound difference between choosing to do nothing and enforced idleness. Enforced idleness leads to a lack of drive and motivation. The patient's self-worth and esteem are lowered, leading initially to powerlessness and despondency and later to extreme apathy.

The excessive use of tranquillising drugs results in lethargy and drowsiness, further diminishing the individual's capacity for self-care and expression. The development of side-effects such as tremors further limits the capacity for occupation and care.

Hierarchical staff structures create a climate of dominance and oppression. Paradoxically the group who should be given the highest priority, i.e., the patients, are found on the lowest level of this power pyramid. The next level is taken up by staff with the least experience and skills, yet with responsibility for the greatest degree of involvement with the client group. This inversion of the power pyramid militates against change and the development of therapeutic programmes of rehabilitation and work.

Options A, B and D: All include fixed meal and work times which do not necessarily lead to institutionalisation. Many people have by necessity to structure and order their day around working times. Fixed rigid routines which affect all of a patient's life, however, are detrimental to the maintenance of individuality.

4. The institutionalised patient can be readily identified from his behaviour and appearance.

Option B is the correct response. All of the descriptions could be applied to the institutionalised patient.

A characteristic behaviour is that of social withdrawal. Such patients often appear to merge imperceptibly with the background and never engage in any meaningful social interactions. Communication may be reduced to almost unintelligible words or short phrases and in extreme cases an elective mutism may be a feature.

The lack of prospects and reduction in skills leads to a failure to plan for the future. In an environment where little changes and basic needs are met, planning for the future becomes meaningless. Dates and days are not recognised as being in any way unique. The past and the future are relinquished for the immediate gratification of the basic needs of the present.

Interest, initiative and motivation are all stifled and apathy is ubiquitous. Such drive as remains is often absorbed in repetitive behaviours, usually concerned with the acquisition of drinks or cigarettes.

Options A, C and D: All include a resentment of harsh orders. In fact patients who have become institutionalised seldom complain about anything. Teasing and brow-beating are tolerated without demure.

5. A base-line is a measure of the extent of a problem and provides a record of the patient's behaviour before the introduction of any treatment.

Option C is the correct response. All of the stated factors provide rationales for making base-line measurements of behaviour.

Observing behaviour and recording the data allows handicaps and deficiencies to be stated in degrees of seriousness. Goal setting and statements of outcomes can then be made before treatment programmes are instituted. It may be noted, for example, that some behaviour is marred by isolated and specific handicaps or deficiencies. Treatment, therefore, should be geared to the correction of those specific areas rather than the adoption of a more global approach. The effectiveness of treatment programmes can only be judged by making comparisons between former and later behaviours. Any change from the base-line level of behaviour indicates the effectiveness or otherwise of treatment programmes. The construction of base-line behaviours provides a record of the full range of problems as they exist and is not dependent on individual bias and selection.

Options A, B and D: All contain analysing the antecedents and consequences of behaviour. This would be undertaken in a full behavioural analysis. The construction of base-lines is concerned simply with the range and scope of the behaviour and not with the wider elements surrounding it.

6. A common model used within behavioural analysis relates to antecedents, behaviour and consequences. The antecedents are those observable features, situations and behaviours which are present immediately before the target behaviour materialises.

Option A is the correct response. A situation could be observed where stamping was linked to those times when the patient sat alone in a corner of the room. This has immediate and obvious implications for the management and modification of that behaviour.

Option B: The general social milieu will have an overall effect on behaviour but does not form part of a behavioural analysis. However, attention does need to be given to these issues in wider management programmes.

Option C: Similarly, isolation from general social norms will have an effect. This can be seen quite dramatically when patients are taken on holiday. Previous bizarre behaviour reduces and is replaced by behaviour judged to be socially acceptable. The return to the institution is accompanied by a resumption of the previous patterns.

Option D: Lowered performance expectations can have a similar long-term effect. These can only be changed by an alteration in the general attitudes towards management of institutionalised patients.

7. A schedule of reinforcement must take account of a number of factors. These include the behaviour to be encouraged or discouraged and the type and timing of rewards.

Option D is the correct response. To be effective the reward should be contingent upon the behaviour to be modified. Rewards which are applied at distant times are unlikely to be effective. This principle underlines the success of gaming machines where rewards, though random, follow immediately upon the gambling behaviour. It is also related to the failure of many to give up smoking for health reasons. In this instance the unpleasant consequences of the behaviour are likely to be experienced far into the future of the action.

Option A: Rewards must be established individually and tailored to the behaviour of a given patient at that moment in time. The principle of equality does not enter into this, though the system should be seen to be fair.

Option B: It has been found that social rewards are the most powerful. The tokens given in some reinforcement schedules may be the vehicle whereby social approval can be expressed.

Option C: A system of behaviour modification should be flexible and changeable, allowing alteration according to client progress or regress. Without this the system would be static and behaviour would alter to a certain level and then remain unchanged.

8. There are a number of techniques which can be utilised to bring about changes in behaviour: these include shaping, prompting, modelling and fading.

Option B is the correct response. Where desirable behaviour is built up in steps which successively approximates to the desired outcome, it is called shaping.

Option A provides a description of modelling. Imitative learning plays a part in the acquisition of many skills. As a technique the nurse or therapist first demonstrates or models a particular sequence of behaviour and then rewards the patient if he successfully copies the behaviour.

Option C   is a description of prompting which can be particularly useful in the early stages of a programme. The patient is helped to perform a behaviour by hints and reminders without the nurse taking over responsibility for the completion of the activity.

Option D   relates to the technique of fading. A process where prompting is gradually removed to the point where the patient can perform the behaviour using his own initiative.

9. Social skills refer to the everyday communications, encounters and relationships that people have with each other: the ability to give and obtain information and to express attitudes, opinions and feelings.

Option B   is the correct response. All of the components could form part of a social skills training package.

The making of requests of others is a skill which combines elements of assertiveness and the interpersonal skills of verbal and non-verbal communication. The person must be able to determine what his needs are, and then to assess whether it is fair and right that he should ask others to help him to meet those needs. An assertive strategy and response has to be made which recognises the needs of others whilst still acting towards a fulfilment of the individual's own needs. The mechanics of making the request, using appropriate verbal and non-verbal behaviour completes the skill.

Offering greetings and goodbyes is a skill which some perform with ease and grace; others find it uncomfortable and difficult. Sometimes general difficulty is experienced. Alternatively, the difficulty may be associated with particular situations or certain people. The identification of problem areas and the tailoring of training to meet those specific needs is important.

Making eye contact is an element which is present in most social encounters. Exercises and structures can be introduced which enable clients to identify problems in this area and practise more effective behaviours. Further elements of non-verbal behaviour which have an influence in relating to others can also be focussed upon.

Options A, C and D: Include looking after hygiene and grooming which fall into the area of self-care. These are important to consider in an overall programme but not necessarily in a social skills training group. Failures to meet acceptable standards of dress and cleanliness may be identified in a social skills training programme; the rectification, however, would be more appropriate to a group involved in learning self-care. It may be decided, of course, to widen the aims of a training group, encompassing, for example, social, personal, domestic amd leisure skills.

Essay questions

1. Jacob Goldstein has been resident in a long-stay ward for 20 years. He tends to isolate himself on the ward and shouts abuse at anyone who approaches him. He hoards rubbish in his pockets and bedside locker, and seldom engages in any constructive activity.

   A What factors may have contributed to the development of this behaviour and be responsible for its continuation?   40%

   B Describe a programme of care which would enable Jacob to engage in more productive and effective behaviours.   60%

2. It is proposed that a social skills training programme be organised as part of a rehabilitation experience.

   A Describe what is meant by social skills training.   30%

   B Outline a programme of social skills training which could help patients to develop their skills in social exchanges and communications.   70%

3. You are working on an integrated rehabilitation ward with a group of patients who have been in hospital for many years. A holiday is being planned for 12 of these patients to be resident in a small guest house at a seaside resort.

   A How should the patients be selected to take part in this venture?   30%

   B Describe a programme which would enable the patients to derive maximum advantage from the holiday.   40%

   C What difficulties may be experienced by the group whilst on holiday?   30%

Specimen answer

1. A A number of general factors associated with life in a psychiatric hospital may
have contributed to the development of Jacob's behaviour.

In many wards housing long-stay patients, there is an expectation and
acceptance of bizarre and strange behaviours. Outside the institution these
behaviours would be responded to by the application of some social sanction.
Inside the institution they are often condoned. This 'mad' behaviour can be
learned and reinforced.

Internal controls become lessened, the patient engaging in strange ways
without inhibition.

Specific antecedents of Jacob's behaviour may include a lack of structure
and stimulation. It may be observed that Jacob engages in collecting rubbish
when he is left alone without occupation. Similarly it may be apparent that he
only verbally abuses people who invade his physical space, or make demands
and requests of him.

Factors contributing to the continuation of his behaviour include
reinforcement by either giving or withdrawing attention. His hoarding may
result in staff paying attention to him by changing his clothes or showing
amusement at his collections. His verbal abuse may serve to keep others
away: he can thereby avoid treatment programmes.

B A programme of care would need to commence with a full behavioural
analysis. Jacob's behaviour, and its antecedents and consequences, should
be fully recorded. From this, a list of behavioural handicaps and deficiencies
can be determined. Base-line observations should be noted in order to
determine the effectiveness of any treatment schedules.

The planning would need to take account of the different behaviours.
Behavioural handicaps could be reduced, often by reinforcement, whilst
behavioural deficiencies respond to teaching, modelling and instruction.

The antecedents and consequences of Jacob's behaviour should be taken
into account and the environment structured to modify these. An improved
structure could be organised for the day, with appropriate rewards for Jacob's
involvement. Giving him some personal possessions may reduce his need to
hoard rubbish. Verbal abuse should be discouraged and Jacob should be
given rewards and reinforcement for other more acceptable social
behaviours.

His withdrawal, isolation and obvious mistrust of others should receive
attention. A consistent, friendly approach should be instituted, initially on a
one-to-one basis. Activities which provide a relatedness without threat, such
as an accompanied walk, could be engaged in. As Jacob develops more trust,
other people could gradually be introduced into the relationship.

Specific techniques of instruction modelling and shaping should be applied
to areas of skills deficit. Reinforcement schedules should be organised to
reduce behavioural handicaps.

Attention must be given to the general social milieu. Staff attitudes and expectations are important. Change should be accommodated gradually, all staff and patients being fully involved in any decisions. Defensive behaviours against change should be openly confronted but in a manner which is supportive.

Evaluation needs to be carried out frequently. Reference to base-line and subsequent observations allows for estimation of improvement or regression. Changes in plans may need to be made according to Jacob's responses, and the programme should aim at being dynamic rather than static.

Answer guides

2. A Social skills training refers to the achievement of competences in the communication and encounters of everyday life: the ability to give and obtain information, make and refuse requests and to express one's needs whilst respecting the needs of others. It is most often undertaken in a small group setting with a trainer or facilitator.

   B A social skills programme dealing with communication could include:
   — assessment of problem areas by interview, observation, questionnaire
   — goal-setting, formulation of objectives
   — development of an understanding of a skilled social performance
   — breaking down a performance into sub-skills
   — practice skills of social encounters with emphasis on verbal and non-verbal communication
   — simulations and role play of social encounters
   — structured group work concentrating on awareness, disclosure and feedback
   — identifying opportunities for practice and support during same
   — exploring feelings relating to achievement or non-achievement, encouraging expressions of cohesiveness and support within the group
   — evaluating progress and planning further sessions.

3. A Selection should be based on:
   — total numbers of patients to go, age range and sex
   — facilities available at venue, skills required
   — staff availability and range of skills
   — patient's level of intellectual, physical, emotional and social skills.
   — motivation and possible benefits of the experience
   — appropriateness to the individual's rehabilitation programme
   — economic factors, affordability.

B Benefit could be increased by:
   — early discussions, allaying of fears, increasing motivation
   — sessions to identify and work on skill deficits
   — involvement in planning holiday and preparation
   — group discussion around holiday venue, things to do and see
   — holiday group to spend time together, engaging in outside visits.
C Difficulties could occur with:
   — individual patients: change in mental or physical state, fears and anxieties, inability to accommodate change
   — the holiday group: arguments and disagreements, conflicting needs
   — staff problems in relationships: with each other or patients due to proximity
   — complaints from managers, other guests
   — untoward occurrences, accidents.

13. Loss of contact with reality associated with confusion

Mrs Elsie Potter is 82 years of age and is at present resident in a psychogeriatric assessment unit. Her medical diagnosis is senile dementia or organic brain syndrome.

Her husband died 3 years ago and whilst the family provide some support, things have become increasingly difficult to manage over the past year. During this time she has been supervised and helped by the community psychiatric nurse. Eventually, however, she became a danger to herself and was admitted to hospital.

Shortly after admission her confusion increased. This was accompanied by agitation and she appeared distressed. She later settled within the unit and her agitation and confusion improved. However, she has difficulty in communicating and needs assistance in carrying out some activities of daily living. Her short-term memory is poor and she exhibits a lack of emotional control.

Multiple choice questions

1. Which one of the following groups contains factors which could all have increased Mrs Potter's confusion upon admission?
   A Removal of familiar objects, provision of structured routines and increase in stimulation.
   B Provision of structured routines, increase in stimulation and strange new surroundings.
   C Increase in stimulation, strange new surroundings and removal of familiar objects.
   D Strange new surroundings, removal of familiar objects and provision of structured routines.

2. Which one of the following activities is likely to prove most difficult for Mrs Potter to relearn?
   A Taking responsibility for her own grooming and hygiene.
   B Performing domestic activities.
   C Planning for future events.
   D Using domestic appliances and machines.

3. Which one of the following interventions is likely to be of benefit to Mrs Potter in structuring her day?
   A Offer a number of choices of activity.
   B Engage in competitive games and pastimes.
   C Encourage decision-making which is challenging.
   D Plan activities which lead to success.

4. Which one of the following groups contains nursing approaches which would all help this patient's understanding?
   A Say one thing at a time, speak slowly and clearly and avoid complex sentences.
   B Speak slowly and clearly, avoid complex sentences and deliver the statement in a number of different ways.
   C Avoid complex sentences, deliver the statement in a number of different ways and say one thing at a time.
   D Deliver the statement in a number of different ways, say one thing at a time and speak slowly and clearly.

5. Which one of the following nursing actions is appropriate if the patient persistently responds with nonsensical statements?
   A Accept the response.
   B Persist until a correct response is given.
   C Confront the patient with the mistake.
   D Ignore incorrect statements.

6. Which one of the following groups contains interactions which would all help to gain this patient's attention in order to improve communication?
   A Shake the patient's arms and shoulders, address by name and approach from front.
   B Address by name, approach from front and make eye contact.
   C Approach from front, make eye contact and shake the patient's arms and shoulders.
   D Make eye contact, shake the patient's arms and shoulders and address by name.

7. Which one of the following groups contains nursing actions which would all help to maximise Mrs Potter's independence?
   A Prepare activities to decrease mistakes, offer a full explanation and then leave to complete in own time, and ask to do one thing at a time.
   B Offer a full explanation and then leave to complete in own time, ask to do one thing at a time, and stay and prompt if necessary.
   C Ask to do one thing at a time, stay and prompt if necessary, and prepare activities to decrease mistakes.
   D Stay and prompt if necessary, prepare activities to decrease mistakes, and offer a full explanation and then leave to complete in own time.

8. Which one of the following groups contains interventions which would all be useful in dealing with Mrs Potter's memory impairment?
   A Adapt new procedures to fit established habits, minimise the complexity of new information and give personalised written notes for future events.
   B Minimise the complexity of new information, give personalised written notes for future events and restrict information to one sensory channel.
   C Give personalised written notes for future events, restrict information to one sensory channel and adapt new procedures to fit established habits.
   D Restrict information to one sensory channel, adapt new procedures to fit established habits and minimise the complexity of new information.

9. Which one of the following provisions may help to reduce nocturnal confusion?
   A Move to a quiet darkened room.
   B Ensure well-lit corridors and annexes.
   C Ensure adequate night-time medication.
   D Move to a bed near to nurse's station.

Answer keys to MCQs

1. The experience of admission is stressful for all and especially the elderly. Sensory impairment and difficulty in assimilating new information leads to increasing confusion. Approaches at this time should aim to lower stimulation and keep things familiar and simple.

   Option C is the correct response. All of the factors may increase confusion upon admission. Any increase in stimulation may lead to sensory overload and inability to perform effectively. Sensory overload results in agitation and distress and a resultant increase in confusion. Strange new surroundings accompanied with hospital noise and bustle can completely disorientate elderly people. Any move from familiar surroundings is upsetting. A move to hospital with its new people, routines and environment may be devastating. The removal of familiar objects helps to complete the disorientation process. Nothing is left of the person's past life and experience to relate to.

   Options A, B and D: All contain the provision of structured routines which can, in fact, help to minimise confusion by simplifying the demands made on the patient.

2. Responsibilities and control should be gradually returned to the patient. However, some activities and functions are relearned with greater difficulty than others.

   Option C is the correct response. Responsibilities requiring higher levels of cognitive functioning such as discrimination, planning and judgement are the most problematic.

   Option A: Generally the more routine the task, the less judgement and discrimination are required. Responsibility for own grooming and hygiene can usually be taken first.

   Option B: Routine tasks in the home or associated with the family are relatively easily resumed.

   Option D: Many patients with impaired intellectual functioning can continue to operate machinery and appliances provided that they are well known. Learning to operate new appliances may be difficult, especially if higher order functions are required.

3. Care should be taken in planning the day to avoid over-stressing the patient which can lead to distress and loss of emotional control. The activities planned should be within the patient's capabilities.

   Option D is the correct response. The activity should have success of the patient as the ultimate goal. She should not be asked to undertake any activity or make decisions which are beyond her competence.

Option A: Making choices from a number of activities involves discrimination and judgement. This can lead to increasing confusion. One idea or task at a time should be introduced.

Option B: Competitive games and pastimes may be over-stimulating. Non-success on the part of the patient also has an effect on others who may confront Mrs Potter with her deficits, thus worsening the situation. Many competitive games also call for turns or planning strategies which she will also find difficult.

Option C: All decision-making should be kept to a minimum and within the patient's capabilities.

4. Verbal communications are best understood when they are kept simple and direct.

Option A is the correct response. All of the approaches would facilitate understanding. Tasks, thoughts and concepts should be introduced one at a time and allowed to be absorbed before others are introduced. Speaking slowly and clearly will also help Mrs Potter to understand the communication. There is no need to raise the voice unless the patient has a hearing difficulty as this can be misconstrued for anger. Care needs to be taken in order not to sound patronising. Speech should be clear and direct. Complex sentences and flowery speech should be avoided as they are confusing.

Options B, C and D: All contain delivering the statement in a number of different ways. Verbal communication may need to be supplemented with visual or non-verbal clues as an aid to remembering the meaning of words. However, restating the message in different words is unlikely to help.

5. Patients who have difficulty in remembering the meaning of words will also have difficulty in finding the right word. They may know what they wish to say and recognise for themselves the difficulty they are experiencing. This can be frustrating and distressing for the patient without it being compounded by the nurse.

Option B is the correct response. Gently persisting and staying with Mrs Potter until she is able to convey her message will do much to allay frustration. Where patients are unable to communicate verbally, then they may resort to acting out behaviours such as yelling, throwing things, pushing and scratching. Listening carefully to both content and also emotional tone can go a long way towards understanding.

Option A: Simply accepting the response does nothing to aid understanding or to help the patient to find ways to communicate her needs.

Option C: The patient is probably well aware of the mistakes. Confronting her with her deficits is likely to lead to increasing anger and loss of emotional control.

Option D: Ignoring the communication is tantamount to dismissing the person. In addition the patient may be trying to communicate important information.

6. Patients with organic brain syndrome have low concentration and attention spans. In order to communicate effectively, nurses need to make sure that what attention is available is directed their way.

Option B is the correct response. All of the interactions would help to gain attention. Addressing the patient by name is a way of making a communication significant and personal as well as being courteous. Using the patient's name also helps in terms of orientation. Approaching the patient from the front gives a chance to prepare Mrs Potter for conversation and rules out surprises. It also helps in establishing eye contact which improves communication.

Options A, C and D: All contain shaking the arms and shoulders which is likely to shock the patient. This may be misinterpreted and provoke an aggressive response. The anxiety caused by the shock would also make further interaction difficult. Some degree of physical contact can help to gain attention, such as putting a hand on the person's arm or hand, but it should never be over-intrusive.

7. The maximising of independent activity should be a prime consideration in the planning of nursing care. The way in which activities are presented and structured has a big effect on the patient's capacity for independent achievement.

Option C is the correct response. All of the actions would be helpful. One task only should be introduced at any one time in order to avoid confusion. Showing the patient, step-by-step, is better than giving a lot of information at one time. Prompting and physically guiding a patient's movements may also be helpful. Activities should be prepared and presented with a view to minimising the possibility of errors and maximising success. For example, clothes can be set out in the order of dressing or routines performed in familiar ways and patterns.

Options A, B and D: All contain giving full information and then leaving to complete in own time. If full information is given all at once, then this cannot be retained and merely leaves patient's anxious and ill at ease. Leaving them to complete an activity gives no consideration to shortened attention and concentration spans. Together the two nursing actions are likely to lead to patient's wandering around agitated and half dressed or other activities being half-completed.

8. Memory impairment is a common feature of organic brain syndrome or senile dementia. Some of the effects of this can be reduced by careful planning.

   Option A is the correct response. All of the interventions would be helpful. Fitting any new routines into established habits will help the patient to adjust to them by taking into account preserved functions. Minimising the complexity of new information by speaking simply and clearly and introducing concepts and tasks one at a time will help. Providing an aide memoire for future events and circumstances is also helpful.

   Options B, C and D: All contain restrict information to one sensory channel. Verbal information often needs to be supplemented by visual clues such as gestures or photographs/symbols. Colour codings and large visual displays can help in orientation.

9. Nocturnal confusion is a common symptom of organic brain syndrome but some of its effects can be minimised by carefully structuring the environment.

   Option B is the correct response. Many patients awake in the night with a desire to go to the toilet. The sensory deprivation and loss of visual clues can lead to increasing confusion at this time. Ensuring that corridors and annexes are well lit can help to reduce this disorientation.

   Option A: A quiet darkened room may be initially restful but upon awakening the lack of sensory input will heighten confusion.

   Option C: Sleeping tablets should be used with care with elderly people as they can further depress brain functioning. Comfort measures to facilitate sleep are a better alternative.

   Option D: Moving the patient to a bed near the nurse's station will improve supervision but the movement and noise will be disturbing.

Essay questions

1. Mrs Elsie Potter, aged 82 years, is admitted to a psychogeriatric assessment unit with a provisional diagnosis of senile dementia.

   A Describe the nursing assessment that may assist in determining Mrs Potter's level of cognitive functioning.   25%

   B Describe how senile dementia may interfere with Mrs Potter's ability to meet her physical needs.   25%

   C Describe a nursing care programme which would ensure that these needs are met.   50%

2. Mrs Elsie Potter, aged 82 years, has been a widow for the last 3 years.

   For the past 12 months she has been supported in her home by the community psychiatric nurse. Recently she has become increasingly confused and disorientated necessitating admission to hospital. She has a short-term memory impairment.

   A What observations could the nurse make to distinguish the normal from the pathological features of ageing?   40%

   B Describe a programme of reality orientation appropriate for Mrs Potter.   60%

3. Mrs Elsie Potter, aged 82 years, has recently been admitted to a psychogeriatric assessment unit.

   Shortly after her admission she became increasingly confused and agitated. Her vision and hearing are impaired and her mobility is decreased.

   A Discuss the factors which could have led to this deterioration in functioning.   30%

   B Describe the nursing management which may help to minimise this type of disturbance.   70%

Specimen answer

1. A Changes in cognitive functioning are a predominant feature in senile
dementia and can be determined in a number of ways. Firstly, information
from other people, such as the family and general practitioner, will give a
picture of deteriorating performance. This will involve processes such as
memory, concentration and judgement. Judgement is a complex intellectual
exercise and failures will quickly become evident in all areas of the patient's
life.

Secondly, a structured interview with the patient can be used to ascertain
problems of understanding and communication. Memory-related questions
can be asked and simple tests of concentration and attention given.

Thirdly, observation of the patient in novel areas will give some idea of her
levels of memory and orientation. Responses to new situations and people,
or to familiar people in new roles and situations, are particularly revealing.
Some assessment of powers of judgement can be made by observing her
activities around the ward: whether she cares for herself appropriately or
relates socially in acceptable ways.

B Changes in cognitive functioning will affect Mrs Potter's ability to meet
physical needs in a number of ways.

Most importantly, judgement will be impaired, and the patient may put
herself at risk and cause accidents resulting in physical damage. She may fail
to take necessary precautions and safeguards, leaving herself short of
essential supplies. Memory loss will have a profound effect on her ability to
look after herself. In new situations she is likely to be lost and unable to
attend to needs such as feeding and elimination. Nocturnal confusion will
interfere with sleeping, whilst anxiety and agitation will impair her chances of
rest and relaxation. Problems with language and understanding will make it
difficult for her to express her needs to others. Appearance and hygiene are
likely to be affected at an early stage due to impairment of judgement and
memory.

C If Mrs Potter is suffering from marked or severe dementia, then her ability to
perceive and to meet her physical needs is minimal. At this time she needs
others to take the responsibility for her physical care. This may include
actually washing, feeding or toileting her. Alternatively, staying with her to
prompt, guide and offer behavioural supervision of her activities may be
sufficient. Although physically capable of fulfilling her needs, she may need
step-by-step direction regarding how and when to fulfil them. The nurse
should recognise that Mrs Potter is unable, rather than unwilling, to perform
these functions.

Such a patient has a low tolerance to either internal or external change, and
relatively small changes can produce profound effects. Ensuring a stable
temperature and environment and looking after the patient's nutritional and
safety needs are essential. The prevention of injuries, particularly those which
immobilise, is an important nursing intervention. Behavioural changes may

signify a change in the patient's physical state. Nursing assessment is critical in determining the presence of physical illness, as Mrs Potter may be unable to perceive or communicate her problems.

The patient's physical safety requires some consideration. Patients who are disorientated often wander away if they are not continuously supervised, and thus put themselves at risk from the hazards of the outside environment. Such patients are also at risk from inflammable and toxic materials and these need to be safely stored and used.

The patient's level of physical arousal needs to be kept at reasonable levels as high arousal leads to increasing delirium. Simplifying and structuring the environment and reducing stimulation are important nursing strategies.

Agitation and delirium may lead Mrs Potter to interfere with the lives of others, causing anger and frustration. Other patients may react aggressively towards such interference and push or hit out causing injury. Nursing programmes should accommodate this by constant monitoring and supervision.

Answer guides

2. A The features of normal ageing can be differentiated from pathological changes on a number of dimensions:

	Normal ageing	Pathological changes
Physical	Gradual decline in dexterity and mobility Some sensory impairment Slowing of response	Paralysis Gross tremors Deafness Blindness
Intellectual	Difficulty in learning new tasks Failing memory Forgetfulness Shorter attention and concentration	Confusion Disorientation Gross memory deficit Wandering
Social	Limiting of social contact Self-centred and demanding Questioning of others' motives	Isolation Paranoid and aggressive Conflict with family, friends
Emotional	Flat or increased response to situations Pessimism Acceptance of death	Emotional liability Lack of emotional control Morbid outlook Suicidal thoughts

B A two-fold approach should be implemented:
   (i) General organisation and management of the ward:
      — provide orientating stimuli: night-lights, calendars, clocks, familiar objects, notices, colour codes
      — orientate in communication: where, who, when, what is expected
      — protect from excessive or confusing stimuli: clear, direct communication; restrict staff numbers; limit duration or numbers of visitors.

(ii) Specific small group work:
 — awareness of self and others
 — practice in recall, concentration, attention
 — communicating with others
 — discussion of current events and topics of interest.

3. A A number of factors operating together may have caused a sudden deterioration in functioning:
 Anxiety and arousal:
 — fear of unknown, of strange procedures
 — lack of understanding for admission
 — fear of long-term consequences
 — confusing and bewildering over-stimulation.
 Unfamiliar environment:
 — lack of familiar objects and memory cues
 — strange bedroom and structures.
 Unfamiliar people:
 — loss of family, friends
 — presence of many others, i.e., patients and staff
 Unfamiliar routines:
 — meals, sleeping, recreation times
 — rigid, inflexible arrangements.

   B Nursing management should address the problems listed above:
 Anxiety and arousal:
 — frequent explanations of what is happening
 — clear, simple, direct communication
 — time to express and explore feelings
 — restrict sensory inputs, use key workers.
 Unfamiliar environment:
 — encourage personal belongings
 — frequently orientate to environment
 — provide night-lights.
 Unfamiliar people:
 — encourage family to visit and provide some care
 — restrict number of staff.
 Unfamiliar routines:
 — adjust new routines and learnings to familiar structures
 — take account of past experience
 — individual care plans.